NO LONGER PROPERTY OF
SEATTLE PUBLIC LIBRARY

INSIDE THE HOT ZONE

INSIDE THE HOT ZONE

A SOLDIER ON THE FRONT LINES

OF BIOLOGICAL WARFARE

Mark G. Kortepeter, MD, MPH
Colonel, U.S. Army (Ret.)

Potomac Books
AN IMPRINT OF THE UNIVERSITY OF NEBRASKA PRESS

© 2020 by Mark G. Kortepeter

All rights reserved. Potomac Books is an imprint of the
University of Nebraska Press.
Manufactured in the United States of America.

Library of Congress Cataloging-in-Publication Data
Names: Kortepeter, Mark, author.
Title: Inside the hot zone: a soldier on the front lines of
biological warfare / Mark G. Kortepeter, MD, MPH, Colonel,
U.S. Army (Ret.).
Description: Lincoln: Potomac Books, an imprint of the
University of Nebraska Press, [2020]
Includes bibliographical references and index.
Identifiers: LCCN 2019016101
ISBN 9781640121423 (cloth: alk. paper)
ISBN 9781640122765 (epub)
ISBN 9781640122772 (mobi)
ISBN 9781640122789 (pdf)
Subjects: LCSH: Kortepeter, Mark. | Biological warfare—
Research—United States. | U.S. Army Medical Research
Institute of Infectious Diseases. | Bioterrorism—
Prevention—History—21st century. | Physicians—United
States—Biography.
Classification: LCC UG447.8 .K67 2020 | DDC 358/.38—dc23
LC record available at https://lccn.loc.gov/2019016101

Set in Arno Pro by Mikala R. Kolander.

Dedicated to my parents, Carl Max and Cynthia Kortepeter, and to my uncle and aunt, Paul and Martha Schmidt, who served as my role models for how to live and work.

Be sober-minded; be watchful. Your
adversary the devil prowls around like a
roaring lion, seeking someone to devour.
    —1 Peter 5:8 ESV

Without a measureless and perpetual
uncertainty, the drama of human life
would be destroyed.
    —Winston Churchill

CONTENTS

Biodefense Solutions to Protect the Nation

—USAMRIID motto

In 1998 the army transferred me to USAMRIID [pronounced YOU-SAM-RID], the U.S. Army Medical Research Institute of Infectious Diseases—the army's biological weapon defense laboratory. USAMRIID's picturesque setting nestled below the Catoctin Mountains at Fort Detrick, Maryland, belies the important germ-warfare defense work ongoing there since the 1950s Cold War era and continuing today against bioterrorism threats.

When I arrived as a junior public health physician and army major, I had no idea that by the time I left as a colonel, I would be pulled into the maelstrom of numerous nationally significant infectious disease crises. I spent seven and a half years inside USAMRIID, affectionately nicknamed the "Hot Zone," after *The Hot Zone*, Richard Preston's bestseller about the institute's discovery of a new species of Ebola virus. Those seven and a half years would be the most exciting of my twenty-seven-plus years wearing the army uniform.

In 1998 the old guard from the former United States' *offensive* bioweapons program (closed in 1969) had moved on. Our mission was bio*defense*. It was an amazing time. The vibrant institute was in its heyday in the afterglow of U.S. success in the first Gulf War and held a unique niche as the nation's go-to place for all things related to biodefense. In an era of openness, knowledge sharing, and relative "innocence," our scientists developed new treatments, vaccines, and diagnostics to thwart potential adversaries like the Soviet Union and Iraq, which might threaten our forces and the nation with deadly infectious pathogens. It was challenging. It was exciting. We were a "family." As with any family, we had our differences and scientific disagreements, but we worked through them and took care of one another inside and outside the lab.

Our world changed after the September 11, 2001, terrorist bombings and the anthrax letter attacks that followed. As quickly as the Berlin Wall went up, a tall black fence grew around us, reminiscent of the Cold War "behind the fence" era of the old offensive biological weapons program. The folksy security guards who watched over our staff late into the night were replaced by a cadre of police armed with pistols, sniper rifles, and 24/7 video monitors. New regulations for enhanced safety and security and nonstop inspections by external agencies bumped science down a notch in priority. In our finest hour, while supporting the nation after the anthrax attacks, our colleagues were targeted as criminal suspects, and one scientist tragically took his own life. Some scientists, frustrated by the constant scrutiny and changing regulations, voted with their feet and left the institute, thus extending USAMRIID's legacy to other burgeoning containment laboratories across the country.

During the period I describe in this book, I moved from the lecture hall to the role of department chief, to the battlefield, to inside the Biosafety Level 4 maximum-containment lab, and finally to the front office. Along the way I played multiple roles as I gained military rank and position: from containing the pathogens and the illnesses they cause, to containing the daily crises, to containing the media explosion and other fallout from crises.

Having read enough narratives by others about what we do, I thought it was time for someone who has walked the halls to tell USAMRIID's side of how certain newsworthy events unfolded. The stories are real, but they could easily serve as plotlines in popular fiction or Hollywood thrillers. Many crises challenged and frightened us, as we didn't know what would come next or how each would end, but we faced each one and made the best decisions we could with the little information available at the time.

Developing countermeasures against deadly pathogens doesn't happen in a weekend, a year, or sometimes not even in a lifetime. It requires years of dedication by determined scientists. I hope the stories I share convey USAMRIID's unique role as a nexus for national response to infectious disease crises and the vital work of my colleagues who toil away daily in the nation's defense, largely unrecognized, and sometimes at their own peril. They are the unsung heroes, and USAMRIID remains critical for the national defense against germ weapons because of them.

Unfortunately, for the sake of crafting a story, I can't include everyone involved or every challenge. The events I describe are seen through the lens of many elapsed years, but I have done my best to fact check them with notes, emails, media reports, and interviews with colleagues. Any mistakes of recollection are mine.

So here I present an insider's perspective depicting the dangers, the drama, the fear, the frustrations, the irony, and the uncertainty encountered as a physician in the role of "Biodefender" in an unusual and occasionally threatening environment.

Join me now as I walk through the "Alamo" security kiosk, past the black fence, up the sidewalk to a two-story tan brick building into a different world—my world—inside the "Hot Zone."

Exposure

FEBRUARY 11, 2004

Around five o'clock on a cool, cloudy evening, a petite, strawberry-blond woman in her late twenties went to work at a research institute on Fort Detrick, Maryland, an army base thirty minutes north of the nation's capital.

She told colleague Dianne Negley in the hallway that she was heading into the lab for a short time. In a locker room for a Biosafety Level 4 (BSL-4) laboratory, the highest level of lab containment, she performed the usual entry ritual. She changed out of her street clothes, removed her watch and wedding ring, and donned scrubs and socks. She passed from the "cold" side locker room that was free of any infectious pathogens into a "warm" side staging area where she taped on gloves, inserted ear plugs, and stepped into an encapsulating, blue, airtight "space" suit with an attached second set of gloves. After pulling the thick sealing zipper from her shoulder down across her front and snapping an air hose into a suit valve, she felt a cool hiss of air spray on her face and neck. As air filled the suit, she puffed up like the Michelin Man; then she walked through a series of airtight doors and entered the "hot" side of a government lab containing the deadliest infectious disease agents on the planet.

Kelly Warfield held a PhD in molecular virology, was an experienced scientist, an army wife, and the mother of a three-year-old boy. Someone who saw her at the grocery store and didn't know what she did for a living might mistake her for a schoolteacher. She worked as a postdoctoral researcher at the United States Army Medical Research Institute for Infectious Diseases (USAMRIID) testing experimental treatments for Ebola virus infection. Known to those in the field as

"YOU-SAM-RID," or simply "rid," it is, more or less, the Pentagon of biodefense—the nation's premier research institute developing medical countermeasures against germ-warfare pathogens. Set behind a tall, reinforced black fence, with tan exterior walls and narrow windows, it looks more like a prison than a research center. Numerous laboratory airflow intake and exhaust pipes that penetrate the flat roof provide a clue to the trained observer of the specialized laboratory capabilities and scientific activities occurring inside.

Kelly entered BSL-4 lab suite AA-5 to check on ten mice she had infected with Ebola virus two days earlier in her search for a cure. One of the most feared infectious pathogens, Ebola kills up to 90 percent of its victims. After ensuring she had adequate air filling the space suit, she unhooked herself from the air hose and waddled down the central white cinder-block corridor dotted with laboratory equipment, video monitors, and multiple coiled yellow air hoses hanging like giant Slinkys from the ceiling.

At the end of the corridor, Kelly pushed open a door to enter the animal room, and she pulled a container of mice off a metal rack. She placed the mice in a beaker inside the laboratory biosafety cabinet (a "hood"), where she could work with them safely. As she studied the animals, none of the mice showed any signs of illness yet. It was still too early. Even so, the virus was already multiplying rapidly inside their bodies.

Kelly sat in front of the bench-level hood, protected by a glass shield while her hands worked inside. One by one, Kelly picked up the mice, flipped them belly-up in her left hand, and injected an immune globulin preparation using a syringe with a thin, twenty-five-gauge needle. It was routine work, something she had done thousands of times before, always with slow and careful hands. As she prepared to inject the fifth mouse, it twitched in her hand, kicking the needle a few millimeters off its precise trajectory. In the flash of a millisecond, she had no time to adjust to avoid disaster. The needle arced downward to the left, pierced through two layers of gloves, and grazed the fleshy heel of her left thumb, just below the joint.

She felt no pain. For a moment she wondered whether the needle had even broken the skin. But when she squeezed her thumb, a tiny dot of blood welled up through the layers of gloves. Just a tiny scratch, but it was as lethal as a hand grenade. That syringe had contained some nonspecific control antibody, not the disease agent. Nevertheless, the needle had been inside four Ebola-infected mice. Her gut plunged like a free-falling elevator, and she shouted,

"*FUCK! FUCK! FUCK!*"

But with the hiss of the air flowing into her suit, alone in the silence of the airtight lab, no one could hear her scream.

Did the needle carry enough virus particles to infect her? It only takes a few to start the cascade that could kill. Kelly knew about the deadly horror that might be coming. She also knew there was no effective treatment. During the first week after infection, the virus launches a clandestine attack on your lymph nodes, bone marrow, spleen, and liver. Around the eighth day, the infection emerges, plummeting your energy and skyrocketing your temperature. Everything aches—your head, your muscles, your joints. Bloodshot lines snake across your eyes, and a spotty red rash grows on your skin like poppies in a field. Your appetite plunges. Over the next several days, your stomach and bowels open above and below, expelling liters and liters of fluid. Blood trickles from your nose and mouth like drips from leaky faucets and oozes from wherever needles penetrate your skin. You are in the thick of Ebola virus disease or hemorrhagic fever. Delirium comes calling as a blessing in disguise to veil your mind from the inevitable end. As your blood pressure bottoms out, your kidneys shut down, and you enter a death spiral.

The shock of the event may have briefly disconnected Kelly's perception of reality. Despite the impact a momentary delay in decontaminating the wound might have on her possible survival, she went into autopilot, tidying things up, meticulously putting all the needles away in a Ziploc bag. Next, she got up and put the mouse cage back in place, not realizing in her daze that she had left some mice in the beaker in the biosafety cabinet.

From there Kelly moved quickly to the decontamination shower, where warm water and a chemical mist sprayed on her suit from nozzles above and all around her. She doused her suit repeatedly with water and chemicals and then aborted the shower's usual seven-minute cycle early. Leaving a trail of water dripping off the suit and puddling on the floor, she unzipped and dropped the suit to the floor and tore off her gloves. Then she called Dianne, whom she had seen earlier in the hallway, but she got an answering machine.

Her second call reached Lisa Hensley, another experienced BSL-4 researcher. "Lisa, this is Kelly. I've had a needle-stick accident. I need you to come down." Kelly then grabbed the emergency bite kit next to the shower door and scrubbed her wound raw with antiseptic.

When Lisa received the distress call, she rushed down to the lab and in her haste was still pulling on her scrubs when she entered the lab's "warm" side. The faces of two other colleagues appeared at the window of the airlock door to assist. Lisa and Kelly left together and flew through the personal shower into the locker room, but a glitch in the electronic sensor failed to trigger the locker-room exit door to open. So they pushed the emergency exit button and broke out of the lab, setting off the institute alarm.

As they hurried through the darkened hallways en route to the clinic past flashing lights with alarm bells ringing, word of the accident spread quickly. Colleagues emerged from offices and labs to follow them, like the Pied Piper, across the institute to the clinic, where my path would intersect with Kelly's for the first time.

•••

That same day in 2004, I was finishing up work in the clinical wing of USAMRIID. It had been a quiet Wednesday, filled with the usual administrative tasks of running the Division of Medicine: chairing lengthy meetings, preparing briefings, reviewing research studies, and dealing with tons of email. I looked forward to going home early—a welcome change from the usual late nights in the office. That would not happen.

Now into my third year as the medicine chief, I oversaw the institute's program to protect and vaccinate lab workers, basically to keep them from being infected by the pathogens they studied. Our scientists conducted research on anthrax, plague, tularemia, Ebola, and many other biological weapon threats, developing and testing vaccines and treatments against them in animals like mice, rabbits, guinea pigs, and monkeys. Anyone stepping foot inside the labs came through us for a rigorous initial evaluation, after which they received recommended vaccines and annual physical examinations.

I had a nice corner office at the end of a long, white-tiled corridor, complete with its own bathroom, narrow window, large mahogany desk, and a beat-up white love seat turned gray with use. I left my office for a meeting and headed toward the nurse's station at the opposite end of the hall, walking past brown corduroy-covered walls interspersed between the offices. As I approached the front of the clinic, a young virologist rushed around the corner, breathless. The words she blurted out made me freeze: "We have an Ebola exposure in the lab!"

I felt like someone had kicked me in the stomach. As the physician in charge, my mind immediately raced through the enormous implications. A member of the lethal filovirus family, Ebola is a Risk Group 4 pathogen, a category reserved for the deadliest organisms. We had no countermeasures. No vaccine. No treatments. No "magic bullet."

Nothing.

Envisioning the grisly death so vividly described in *The Hot Zone* and the front-page headlines that would follow, I fought the swell of panic, but reminded myself to ignore my own fears and shift focus to my perspective as a physician. We now had a patient. The patient always comes first. The military has a saying: "When in charge, take charge." I needed to devise a response plan . . . quickly. Our patient deserved that.

We had a small window of time to keep the lid on Pandora's laboratory, a containment lab filled with billions of live microscopic pathogens. With my experience in biodefense and public health, I knew the stakes.

USAMRIID had a special two-bed isolation unit, the only one of its kind in the United States at that time, called the "Slammer." Designed with all the trappings of an ICU (intensive care unit), the Slammer was built precisely for such emergencies in the era of the Apollo moon landings to isolate patients infected with the most dangerous pathogens—even extraterrestrial ones, like the "Andromeda Strain."[1]

Modeled after our Biosafety Level 4 (BSL-4) labs, the Slammer was a negative-airflow suite that sucked air into its three rooms so no germs could escape. Air passed through specialized air filters on the way in and before being released into the environment, and liquid waste passed through a steam sterilizer. Unlucky Slammer "guests" might feel more like prisoners than patients, locked up for weeks in quarantine by doctors wearing space suits, waiting for the disease to strike.[2] No one can better imagine such a lonely, agonizing death than someone who studies Ebola every day.

Feeling an intense wave of fear and dread, I asked the virologist who had conveyed the bad news a couple of quick questions to ensure that this wasn't a false alarm. Then I turned around and walked briskly back down the hall to find Lieutenant Colonel Scott Stanek, an army public health doc, and Colonel Jim Martin, an army infectious disease doc. Scott is tall, thin, with a strong jaw, a calm demeanor, and an avid interest in U.S. military history. Jim is of average height, with short brown hair, a long-distance runner's build, and wire-rimmed glasses that give him a "preppy" appearance. I would need assistance from both because Scott and Jim were in charge of maintaining the physical Slammer space. Most of the Slammer staff worked for me, and my team managed any lab exposures, so I would be in charge of the overall response.

"I think we may have a Slammer admission," I said and gave them a quick run-down of what little I knew—just enough to worry us all. I asked them to make any final preparations of the suite to admit a patient.[3]

I needed more information to determine the severity of this exposure and what measures to take. The institute had a routine process for handling lab exposures, but every crisis came with its own nuances.[4] By this time I had the scars of experience managing lab exposures, usually from the Biosafety Level 2 (BSL-2) or BSL-3 labs—the occasional dropped vial, cut finger, monkey bite, or animal body-fluid splash. Those were routine.

Exposures in BSL-4 were not. The last Slammer admission had occurred back in 1985, nineteen years earlier.

This was a major crisis and the most serious lab exposure of my tenure. Kelly could be the first Ebola victim ever on U.S. soil. No one knew how to treat Ebola, so we would be running blind—while under the scrutiny of the media microscope. It would be a significant test of my leadership.

Physicians are taught to take their own pulse first before they take the patient's when responding to a code blue, a medical term for a cardiac arrest emergency. So I took a deep breath to calm myself and then sought out my clinic chief, Dr. Ellen Boudreau, a pediatrician with expertise working on experimental malaria treatments on the Thai borders. At the time she had at least five years of experience managing laboratory exposures. I knew she would ask the right questions.

Ellen's short gray hair and rosy cheeks match her nurturing personality. She cares for her patients like she would her own children. When I stepped into her office, she was at her desk typing inside a cavern of precariously stacked patient charts, leaning like the Tower of Pisa, ready to topple at any moment. I quietly asked her to do the baseline history and physical exam on Kelly when she arrived.

Understandably, Ellen wasn't too excited, as she thought, *This could be a lethal mistake,* but she accepted the task like a pro.

When Kelly arrived at the clinic, she sat down in the closest office with Denise Clizbe, a nurse who knew her well and often witnessed crises unfolding in the clinic. Looking terrified, like a deer in headlights, Kelly confided that she worried especially about her young son.

Moments later Kelly disappeared into a clinic exam room with Ellen. Kelly was a little teary-eyed and upset with herself. She had concerns that any working mother might have: she couldn't take a break from her research. She couldn't take a break from her family. People depended on her. What was she going to do?

While in the exam room, Kelly put in a call to her husband, Jeremy, an army doctor, who was away in Texas. Jeremy rattled off a series of questions in rapid sequence: "What does this mean?" "What's going to happen?" "What happened to the monkeys when you gave them that virus?"

They were the same questions that she might consider if she allowed herself to think. Overwhelmed, she just handed the phone to Ellen to respond.

Jeremy's questions continued: "What's going on here?" "Do you know what's going on, because I can't believe this is happening, and who are you, and what is your training?" "Are you the right person to take care of my wife?"

Ellen explained that she was a pediatrician. "But I will hand this over to our ID [infectious disease] specialist, Dr. Kortepeter, who is a colonel, and he has military clout," she assured him.

Jeremy seemed content at that point, saying, "I want the best specialists on this."

While Ellen evaluated Kelly in the exam room, all hell broke loose in the clinic. Like relatives arriving at a funeral, physicians, virologists, safety representatives, Kelly's supervisor, the lab suite supervisor, and the USAMRIID deputy commander descended on us from all over the institute, offering their opinions and asking myriad questions.

I had learned from previous mistakes to bring the right people to the table at the beginning in order to shut down any armchair quarterbacking later when they didn't like my decisions. So I ushered about eleven key leaders into a standing meeting crammed into Ellen's freight-elevator-sized office.[5] With only a foot between us, while we argued about possible courses of action, Ellen leaned into the doorway and briefed us on what she had learned. Kelly had sustained a scratch barely visible on her left thumb, but a small amount of mouse blood or body fluids containing Ebola virus could have contaminated the needle.

At peak infection Ebola can reach concentrations of over one hundred million virus particles in a milliliter of blood. That's like cramming the four-hundred-billion-plus stars in the Milky Way Galaxy into a drop of blood. At this early stage, there would be fewer virus particles in the mouse blood, but that might still be enough to start the deadly cascade. Even worse, Kelly was working on the deadliest of the five Ebola species: Ebola Zaire. During outbreaks in the African jungles, up to 90 percent of victims had died. After a needle stick, 100 percent died.[6]

We heatedly debated our possible actions. Should we send her home and monitor her there for three weeks? It had worked previously for lower-risk exposures. The virologists favored that option. But it came with great and obvious risks.

How would we respond if someone in the Institute leaked it to the press? How would the community react if people learned there was an Ebola-exposed patient living among them? We knew the answer. It would set off a firestorm. Also, if Kelly went home, what would we do when she spiked a fever? We would have to transport her back to the Slammer. That would be hard to do quietly.

I envisioned a front-page *Washington Post* photo bomb with Kelly visible inside our clear plastic transportable isolator, like E.T., the extraterrestrial, being wheeled by our Aeromedical Isolation Team in full protective space suits to a waiting Humvee with a police escort past gawking neighbors and rolling CNN cameras. It would be a complete disaster.

The other option, favored by the docs: put Kelly in the Slammer immediately. Although I wanted to side with the virologists, my gut dictated otherwise. On the hospital wards, I had learned to trust my instincts. On the other hand, I was the father of three young boys. I couldn't fathom the thought of saying goodbye to my three-year-old, knowing I might never see him again and face a lonely, horrible death in a week. But I also knew the grave risks. Having Kelly's husband out of state posed additional challenges.

The consensus shifted back and forth a little longer, but as the institute commander's senior physician advisor, I had to make the final call. I interrupted the discussion and said, "I don't feel comfortable sending her home."

This decision pulled the twenty-one-day home quarantine option off the table. We then reconsidered the incubation period, the time between the exposure and when the victim first breaks with a fever. For Ebola it ranges from two to twenty-one days, although most victims spike a fever in about a week. Fortunately, Ebola didn't appear to spread until after someone feels sick. This bought us a little time, because the risk to others should be minimal, at least for a couple of days.

My final recommendation to the commander: let Kelly go home for the night and get her affairs in order. This gave her a chance to say goodbye to her son and find a contingency for her three cats. It was the right thing to do, although I felt some misgivings that my military chain of command and the public might not be so easily convinced when word got out. It also gave us a couple of hours to make final preparations in the Slammer for her admission and time for her husband to get on a plane. This process would not be simple. We would have to build a crisis response team and rip everyone out of their day jobs to assist.

When the meeting broke up, I walked with Kelly slowly down the hallway to my office. There we sat across from each other at my small conference table, and I reviewed the plan with her.[7] My prior experience informing patients that they have cancer or telling family members that their loved one was dying probably helped me with this discussion. Even so, I don't know who was more nervous, Kelly or me, but she appeared to be holding up well. I told her to return the next morning at 8:00 a.m.

Kelly was destined for the Slammer.

INSIDE THE HOT ZONE

Beginnings

....

Kelly's odyssey will continue later, but in the meantime, how the hell did I end up here, keeping the lid on the deadliest virus on the planet in the nation's "Hot Zone"?

Despite my shaking hands and unsettled gut, my years of training and experience up to this point had prepared me well to handle the situation if I trusted my instincts.

I spent my early years in London, Toronto, and Istanbul due to my father's work as a university professor. We moved back to the United States when I entered first grade. Living overseas at a young age gave me an appreciation for other cultures and foreign languages, which would help me later in international work. My parents put a strong emphasis on education and constantly pushed me and my five siblings to achieve. Although money was a frequent stressor, I was incredibly fortunate to have educational opportunities on par with the Kennedys.

My parents tried to peg our future careers based on our respective talents. My eldest brother was the "engineer," the next one the "writer." I was third, the "doctor," because I excelled in math and science. Although I started out wanting to be a scuba diver, I did have an early fascination with medicine, frequently perusing the clear plastic images of the human body in our home edition of the *Encyclopedia Britannica*.

As the shy one in the family's upper tier, I often refereed dinner-table arguments between my more vocal and opinionated older brothers and father. My willingness to listen and be less judgmental would serve me well later as a doctor and a leader.

Although I was shy, I had early independence thrust on me. I showed talent on the violin, so at age twelve I boarded a smoke-filled bus every Sunday for the one-and-a-half-hour ride from New Jersey into New York City for violin lessons. Feeling scared and lonely, I channeled my way through bustling crowds and the subway maze uptown to West Seventy-Third Street. I dreaded the Sunday commute, but the experience gave me skills maneuvering around a city and remaining alert to my surroundings.

Performing for an audience helped me overcome some of my timidity. For two summers I attended the Meadowmount School of Music, a Juilliard-quality summer strings camp in upstate New York, which was attended by the likes of Joshua Bell, Pinchas Zukerman, and Itzhak Perlman. Having accomplished friends, some of whom were already famous, probably helped me later not to be intimidated by army generals.

My violin opened numerous doors for me. Most importantly, I played in a youth symphony that rehearsed at the Lawrenceville School, a prestigious boarding school in New Jersey. My father told me to apply for admission. A timely phone call he made to the director of admissions landed me nearly a full tuition scholarship when another boy backed out. It showed me the importance of chance and timing, but also the value of picking up the telephone to solve a problem.

Lawrenceville challenged me and laid the academic foundation for my future pursuits. During my first year, I decided I wanted to be a high jumper on the track team, so during spring break, I crafted a makeshift high-jump setup by piling two old mattresses on top of each other, building two wooden stands, and buying a piece of bamboo for the cross bar. I spent the break practicing. When I got back to school, the effort paid off. I made the track team. Two years later I won a gold medal in the state championship. This achievement added another lesson for success: persistence. One teacher gave me the ultimate compliment: "Kortepeter is a scholar athlete."

Eventually, I embraced the idea of pursuing medicine. It helped to have a family member to emulate. My uncle was a seasoned cardiologist who had served as a navy doctor with the marines in the Vietnam jungles. While I was in high school, I saw patients with him and watched him conduct treadmill tests and heart catheterizations.

After shadowing my uncle, I wanted to become a cardiologist too. I had multiple "windows" into the heart, hearing its "lub dub" with a stethoscope and watching the squeezing doughnut-shaped muscle and fluttering heart valves open and close with an ultrasound probe. Electrocardiogram tracings on pink graph paper were as confusing as hieroglyphics, but my uncle interpreted them as skillfully as the Rosetta Stone.

I arrived at Harvard overconfident and struggled with mediocre grades my first two years, which knocked my ego down several notches. Working on the side to supplement my scholarship probably didn't help.

In our dorm, my roommate Ed and I chowed down on Korean food made by his mom, while huddling on a threadbare olive-drab couch with other doctor wannabes to view nightly reruns of *M*A*S*H*. We all admired TV army doctor Hawkeye Pierce's surgical skills and compassion, as he and Trapper John cut through an endless stream of blown-up limbs with humor. I was tall, thin, and gangly, like the actor Alan Alda, so one year I dressed up as Hawkeye for my dorm's Halloween party wearing blue scrubs and tinfoil dog tags. The thought of actually joining the army, though, had not yet crossed my mind.

By junior year I had matured. My first job in the library had paid a measly $2.65 an hour, but by junior year I accepted more menial labor cleaning dorm bathrooms in exchange for a raise to $5.15 an hour. Less time working for the same total pay freed up my schedule. I refocused on my classwork, and it paid off, but the earlier years at Harvard had shattered my confidence. I feared I wouldn't get into medical school, and I lost opportunities to compete for prestigious travel scholarships. I resolved that if I *did* get accepted into medical school, I would prove that I deserved it by doing something important to make a larger impact beyond just patient care. I also felt a burning desire for the adventurous travel I missed out on by failing to win the scholarships. Only now, in retrospect, do I realize how strongly my early failures influenced my drive and future pathway.

I was elected vice president/treasurer of my 250-person dorm. The position required me to speak in front of the dorm council, but the real value came from observing my more outgoing friend, Jim, run the council meetings. Learning how to run a meeting would prove to be one of the most valuable skills that I learned in college and applied years later leading different departments and research organizations.

I regained some of my confidence in medical school. I found the work conceptually easier than college. But medical school was a lonely and depressing period, although a close circle of friends made it tolerable. Living on loans, I shared an apartment with four roommates, shivering in a basement room as cold as a meat locker. I strung sheets of plastic around my bed during the winter in a feeble attempt to keep the heat in, generated by my anemic space heater. Every day I feared my rusting Fiat would break down in the heart of the Newark, New Jersey, ghetto while I was driving to school.

One thing Newark did have in abundance, though, was sick patients, which every medical student needs. The bustling emergency room held a nightly chorus of patients dying of sepsis, gunshot wounds, or fungating cancers. The myriad drug overdoses were stacked in the corridors to detoxify rather than being admitted to the hospital.

The seeds of my future interest in infectious diseases were planted on the Newark hospital wards. One of my female African American patients left an indelible impression on me. Deathly ill from pneumonia, feverish, shaking, and coughing up sputum that looked like butterscotch pudding, she couldn't even muster the energy to sit up in bed.

I took a sample of her sputum down to the lab and performed a "Gram's stain." Named after Danish bacteriologist, Hans Christian Gram, it's a simple procedure that even a medical student can do. Start by smearing a drop of sputum on a glass slide, then hold it over a flame for a couple of seconds to "fix" the sputum tightly to the glass. After that pour on some purple dye, followed by iodine, and then watch lines of purple rinse away with a quick squirt of alcohol. Finally, flood the slide with a second, pink stain.

Certain bacteria retain the purple dye in their cell wall, so they appear "Gram positive" (purple) under the microscope. In others the alcohol rinses away the purple dye, so they stain "Gram negative" (pink) instead. This simple distinction drives important treatment decisions, because some antibiotics kill Gram positive and others kill Gram negative bacteria.

When I peered through the microscope at my patient's sputum, I saw the telltale signs of pneumonia: sheets of white blood cells that looked like fried eggs, with purplish single or multi-lobed "egg yolk" nuclei surrounded by grainy pink and purple dotted "egg whites." Lawns of much smaller purple dots came into focus under higher magnification as "lancet" shaped bacteria in pairs—rounded on one end with the other pointy ends kissing. Some bacteria had been gobbled up, like Pac Man, by the white blood cells.

The lancet shape and color were characteristics of *Streptococcus pneumoniae,* or "pneumococcus." Nicknamed "Captain of the men of death," in the pre-antibiotic era, pneumococcal pneumonia had a well-deserved reputation as a feared killer. If she had delayed coming to the hospital one more day, my patient probably would have died. Once my Gram stain demonstrated what she had, choosing the right antibiotic was simple.

After she had received two days of intravenous antibiotics, I watched stunned and elated as my patient got out of bed, like an awakening Lazarus. I couldn't believe that the care I had provided had such an immediate, life-saving impact.

The tiny bacteria fascinated me. They grew and changed color on petri dishes as they coalesced like water droplets or morphed into fluffy, shiny, or slimy globs. Some gave off inviting grape fragrances, while the smell of others turned your stomach like a putrid, dead squirrel. But captured inside the world of the microscope lens, they became beautiful clusters of purple grapes, pink boxcars, or blue safety pins.

Just as I started on the medical wards in 1985, HIV mowed down the Newark intravenous (IV) drug-user population like a field combine. My classmates and I feared we would be the next HIV victims. I drew blood on my patients with bare hands back then because I could feel the puffy elongated shapes of the veins easier, but I spilled blood on my hands more than once when putting in an IV catheter. My roommate once said to me with frightened resignation, "Mark, you know we've all been exposed."

My HIV patients entered the hospital feverish, coughing, and over the next couple of days, their chest x-rays "blossomed" from black to white as if filled with cotton. We watched helplessly as they gasped for breath and suffocated, despite our antibiotics. Feeling chagrined that I couldn't do much for my HIV patients, I moved studying infectious diseases to a back burner. Getting one step closer to becoming the next Hawkeye Pierce became a reality, though, when I realized what a good deal my medical-school roommate had when he was awarded a military scholarship that paid his tuition. I decided to apply, but I had missed the deadlines for the navy and air force programs, so it was complete serendipity that I applied only to the army. Once accepted I signed nervously on the dotted line. Committing to give the army four years after medical school seemed like a lot then, but my attitude changed when I flew to Hawaii my senior year to train at an army hospital for a six-week student rotation.

I arrived in Honolulu the weekend of July 4, a spanking-new "butter bar" second lieutenant (nicknamed for the rectangular bronze insignia on the shoulder) in a crisp green uniform, not even knowing who, or how, to salute. From the moment I got off the plane, heard the chirping birds outside, and was engulfed in the perfumed fragrances of tropical flowers, I knew I had made the right decision.

I couldn't start on the hospital wards without "in-processing," but the administrative offices had closed for the long weekend. So I asked myself, "What to do in Hawaii?" For starters a fellow medical student and I drove east past Diamond Head out to Hanauma Bay, where the ocean side of a burned-out volcano had eroded, leaving a crystal-blue bay teaming with brightly colored tropical fish and coral. We basked in the sun on tatami mats on a white sand beach among Japanese tourists, surrounded by lush green cliffs. My friend turned to me with a grin and said, "Doctor, do you realize you are being paid fifty dollars a day to sit on this beach?" "Wow!" I said. "The army isn't such a bad deal, after all." "It's good to be the king," he laughed, quoting from Mel Brooks's *History of the World*.

When I graduated from medical school in 1988, the army helped me escape as far from Newark as possible and sent me to San Francisco for my transitional internship. When I arrived as a new army captain, on my first day on the hospital wards, my bald, overweight neurology resident, who outranked me as a lieutenant colonel, pulled me outside during his hourly smoke break.

"Here's how this works," he said in between drags on his cigarette. "For this month, basically, you are my dog."

Suppressing my desire to tell him exactly where to shove his cigarette, I did the work for both of us while he smoked away his days. I would stumble out of the hospital at midnight in search of fast food and return early each morning to start over again. The internal medicine guys on call took pity on me when we ran into each other in the radiology suite in the wee hours, and I decided I wanted to be one of them. I wasn't surprised when my resident was later fired for incompetence and banished to a remote army base in Alaska.

My first month as an intern, on a Saturday morning, a petite Asian American pharmacist named Cindy summoned me to the pharmacy to sign a prescription for a patient I was discharging. A year later, before I shipped off for Hawaii, we eloped to City Hall on her lunch break. We hadn't even bought rings yet. We later held our formal wedding in San Francisco, just four days after the 1989 earthquake. Why she decided to hitch a ride with me, I'll never know. Perhaps the earthquake foreshadowed some of the unexpected excitement and challenges to come.

I arrived in Hawaii for the second time in 1989 excited and more than a bit nervous to launch into my internal medicine residency training. Tripler Army Medical Center served as the referral hospital for tens of thousands of military forces stationed throughout the Pacific. Framed by the lush green Koolau Mountains, the coral-colored "pink palace" hospital stares down on Pearl Harbor like a formidable, giant Buddha statue.

My fellow residents-in-training at Tripler had already worked together for a year and probably wondered whether they could trust the "new guy." One morning one of my colleagues was cornered by our attending physicians in a merciless "shark attack" while presenting a case at our daily case conference. Usually, when "blood was in the water," the other residents cowered on the sidelines, lest they become the sharks' next targets. Training through embarrassment seemed juvenile and unnecessary, so I decided to throw a wrench into the process. I was beginning to overcome my timidity and just happened to have a good case that I had not yet presented. When the staff served up my bloodied fellow resident for another meal, I jumped boldly into the fray, offering to present my case instead. My colleague gratefully yielded his place on the stage. My presentation went well.

The next day I was summoned to an "emergency" residents' meeting. As I took my seat in the conference room, the chief resident called me up to the front of the room. As I stood there, surprised and confused, he read off a citation mimicking a military award. "Ladies and Gentlemen, attention to orders."

All the residents stood at attention in unison. The chief resident awarded me the inaugural "Shark Attack" medal, "for demonstrating courage to enter shark-infested waters to save a fellow resident." They pinned a paper badge on my white coat with a red "no sharks" circle and diagonal line overlying a sketch of a shark—a mere strip of paper but more valuable to me than Olympic gold. I had earned the trust and respect of my new colleagues.

While at Tripler, Colonel Joel Brown, an infectious disease doctor and Vietnam veteran, revived my interest in infectious diseases. Tall, with a straight back, shaved head, and imposing military bearing, he enthralled me with exotic-sounding diagnoses, like malaria, dengue fever, leptospirosis, and leishmaniasis, for our patients flown in from all over the Pacific Rim. The idea of working with treatable, as opposed to chronic, diseases, in addition to their link to travel, sold me. I wanted to study infectious diseases like Colonel Brown.

The many nights on call in Hawaii passed by in a blur, but after a couple of months, at around two o'clock one night, I realized how far my medical skills and confidence had advanced. I had just discharged my last patient from the now dark and desolate emergency room. I thought to myself, *I can handle whatever comes in the door.*

In 1992, with my residency training over, Cindy and I shipped off to Fort Bragg, North Carolina. While we were there, our first son, Luke, arrived. I was head of the HIV clinic and continued to be frustrated watching my patients die with only a single medication, AZT, at our disposal. I reassessed my goals. Although I loved my patients, public health offered a chance to prevent future infections, chase down infectious disease outbreaks, and make a bigger impact beyond individual patients. I applied for further training in public health/preventive medicine. After two years at Bragg, I was promoted to major. Then we packed our bags for a year each in Boston and Tacoma, Washington, before we landed at Fort Sill, Oklahoma. There wasn't much there except flat land, pink rubble, tumbleweeds, and tarantulas—and the wind really does come "sweeping down the plains." Armed with a freshly printed public health degree, I ran a health department of fifty people that stretched across three army bases. The work kept me hopping, but I started to build my foundation in leadership running that department.

After two years in Oklahoma, which included a nine-month deployment as the senior public health doctor for the U.S. forces in the Bosnia peacekeeping mission, I requested a transfer to the Walter Reed Army Institute of Research in Washington DC, which develops countermeasures against military infectious disease threats, like dengue fever and malaria. I wanted the chief of Field Studies job, which I hoped would position me to conduct research around the world and fulfill my travel bug. However, one afternoon I received a phone call from a former colleague from Tripler that would have a huge impact on my future. She wanted that same assignment. Would I consider taking her position at USAMRIID instead?

I had toured USAMRIID two years earlier. The place had a fascinating and mysterious aura as the largest biodefense lab in the world. Could this be the opportunity I had waited and trained for?

"Sure," I said, "why not?" A win-win.

Keeping us both happy made it easy for our assignments officer.

Before we left Oklahoma, Cindy and I welcomed son number 2, Sean.

My arrival at USAMRIID in 1998 coincided with a wave of bioterrorism hoaxes popping up around the country like weeds in a garden. I joined the small Operational Medicine Division, with six docs and a mission to "translate the science" of biological weapon defense into practical measures for military docs and nurses. We also served as a national resource for any calls related to bioterrorism. My team developed lectures, wrote articles, and drafted policies on treating biological weapons casualties. We had a unique niche and no shortage of audiences inside and outside the military requesting our expertise. My first task was to write, produce, and cohost a satellite television show on biodefense.

Excuse me? In college, I could barely write a ten-page paper. Now I had to come up with a twelve-hour television script? I dove right in, and to my amazement, I discovered that I had a knack for writing when I wrote about something I liked. Suddenly I was working with international experts. I felt exhilarated as cohost with my colleague Ted Cieslak, dialoguing on-camera in front of thirty-thousand viewers with Dr. D.A. Henderson, leader of the global smallpox eradication campaign, as he read the smallpox script on the teleprompter that *I had written* for him. Without realizing it, like molting an outer skin, I had shed my shyness.

I couldn't believe my good fortune, and I couldn't wait to go to work every day. I had found my niche, was fulfilling my desire to travel by teaching around the world, and believed I was doing important work protecting the nation.

Robert Frost's "The Road Not Taken" has a special meaning for me and my decision to go to USAMRIID:

Two roads diverged in a wood, and I—
I took the one less traveled by,
And that has made all the difference.

I found myself on biodefense preparedness panels and received invitations as a keynote speaker for multiple venues, which would never have happened if I had stayed in internal medicine or general public health.

At one point a former USAMRIID commander invited me to join a workgroup retreat in St. Michaels, Maryland, a tiny town on the Eastern Shore of the Chesapeake Bay. Our task was to generate a list of the top biological weapon threats to the U.S. military. I found myself among a who's who of infectious disease and biodefense experts, which included Dr. Henderson; a couple of former USAMRIID commanders; Bill Patrick, chief of New Product Development for the former U.S. Bioweapons Program; Yellow fever expert Tom Monath; Ebola expert and USAMRIID senior scientist Peter Jahrling; and Ken Alibek, a former leader of the Soviet Union's biological weapons program.

I scanned the room and wondered how I, a junior army public health doc, got invited to the party. Surely someone had made a mistake. Nevertheless, I did my best to disguise my feelings of intimidation, and I realized that I had a lot to contribute. The meeting gave me strong incentive and ambition that someday I might join their ranks as a senior leader and expert in this field. I had found my calling: to protect military personnel and the nation from biological weapons.

My two years in Operational Medicine gave me a good foundation for understanding the diseases and the countermeasures to treat or prevent them. Then, in 2000 the chief of USAMRIID's Medicine Division, a former colleague from Fort Bragg asked me, "How long do you want to write about other peoples' research?"[1]

He recruited me to join the division as his deputy. It was a difficult decision to leave the excitement of Operational Medicine, but I was about to pin on the rank of lieutenant colonel, and I believed the job might bring new opportunities and skills. I would also gain an additional mission, protecting a different kind of hero: the laboratory workers who put themselves at risk every day working with the deadliest infectious pathogens on the planet.

So after a long and jagged road, it was a combination of chance and interest, if not destiny, that led me to Wednesday, February 11, 2004, when my path crossed Kelly Warfield's and the most serious Ebola exposure in the nation in decades. By then I had built a foundation of skills, like layers of a cake, with experience in patient care, field public health, leading a public health department, and bioweapon defense. I was as prepared as I could be in my quest to protect the lab workers, the institute, the military, and the nation against bioweapons, but I would need an additional skill in order to effectively manage Kelly's exposure: crisis management.

I would have multiple opportunities to build on that layered foundation as new crises tested me in the coming years, including the bioweapon challenge hiding just around the corner.

2

Germs as Weapons

....

Whether it's an outbreak of Ebola virus, anthrax, or Zika virus, Mother Nature likes to keep us humble. Infectious diseases have shaped history and brought down empires. When Europeans came to the New World, infections they carried with them, like smallpox and measles, killed more Native Americans than bullets. By some estimates 95 percent of the indigenous population was wiped out by these illnesses.[1]

We witnessed havoc and fear in the United States in 2014–16 when an Ebola outbreak struck an ocean away in West Africa. Just imagine the potential panic from a bioterrorist attack with Ebola inside the United States. Ebola enjoys membership in an exclusive "club" of infectious pathogens with properties that make a "good" bioweapon, but despite its high fatality rate and fear it engenders, Ebola is not the top dog . . . not by a long shot.

Countries continually seek new ways to gain military advantage. Humans have dreamed up chemical and nuclear agents to tip the balance in warfare. Mother Nature gave us the tools for biological (germ) warfare to unleash deadly contagion against our enemies through living organisms or toxins they produce. A germ attack can be executed in multiple ways, depending on an enemy's objectives and sophistication.

Something as simple as human feces or a dead animal carcass can become a weapon if dropped into an enemy's well to contaminate the water supply. Move up one level of sophistication by burying a sharp stake smeared with feces, and you've created a punji stick, a simple weapon used against our forces in Vietnam to pierce a combat boot and cause a horrible, putrefying infection.

Germ warfare jumped to a new level of sophistication in the early twentieth century when the superpowers harnessed microbiology to create new tools of death. The U.S. government officials feared that the Japanese and the Germans had gotten the jump on them and didn't want to fall behind. In 1943 universities and pharmaceutical companies joined the government in a top-secret program to develop germ weapons, which was headquartered at Camp Detrick, Maryland (now Fort Detrick). Other countries joined the germ "arms race," including the United Kingdom, Canada, Japan, and the former Soviet Union. Iraq, Syria, Libya, North Korea, and Iran, all suspected of supporting terrorism, probably also launched their own programs, not only in biological weapons, but also in chemical weapons. The U.S. program conducted elaborate tests to assess the country's vulnerability to a bioweapon attack. Simulant organisms, which were similar to bacterial pathogens but not deadly, were released off the coast of San Francisco, with collection devices arrayed all around the Bay Area that showed that the organisms went far and wide. Another experiment placed a simulant for anthrax in light bulbs that were then shattered on the tracks of the New York City subway. The moving subway cars acted like pistons, pumping the organisms throughout the subway system.

Although they ran different weapons programs on opposite sides of the globe, the Soviets and the Americans selected surprisingly similar pathogens to weaponize and cause diseases such as anthrax, botulism, tularemia, Q fever, and Venezuelan equine encephalitis (vee). Clearly, those agents were selected for their unique properties, but it probably helped that Soviet spies during the Cold War had infiltrated Fort Detrick.

The Soviets also seemed enamored of deadly or contagious agents causing diseases like smallpox, plague, and influenza—yes, the flu! Mother Nature then would do the dirty work of spreading the disease like wildfire, once the Soviets lit the kindling.[2]

The Americans, on the other hand, favored incapacitating weapons. A sick person ties up more people caring for him or her than a dead one. The Americans also considered the advantage of destroying crops and developed wheat stem rust and rye stem rust, because if an army "runs on its stomach," an adversary can't go far if you wipe out its rations.[3] A strike against our cattle or swine populations or wheat fields could destroy large segments of our economy and roil the stock market.

Not every microbe makes a "good" biological weapon for war, but if chosen and released correctly, the right weapon could wipe out enemy forces and possibly determine the outcome on the battlefield. The "best" weapons share some key properties: They survive well and infect efficiently in the air. They grow easily enough to generate large quantities to spray over a battlefield. They are highly infectious, sickening most of their exposed victims, and they shouldn't come back to infect one's own troops, so it helps to develop vaccines against them.

Biological weapons are fickle, though, so timing is everything. The weather must cooperate. You can't unleash an attack in a thunderstorm. A gentle, steady wind is ideal for wafting an airborne weapon toward the enemy—but not too fast, or the aerosol dissipates. Too slow or in the wrong direction, and you miss the target, or it comes back to bite you. The sun degrades most organisms, so better to release them at nighttime for maximizing casualties, when the stealthy night air creates an inversion and hugs the weapon close to the ground and its intended victims.

Bioterrorists may have different requirements, depending on whom they target and whether they seek to kill people, sicken them, scare them, or just make a political statement. They may need smaller amounts than used in warfare to assassinate a political figure, contaminate a salad bar, or kill a neighbor.

Among the thousands of possible microbes, the cast of frightening diseases with the properties that make a "good" bioweapon shrinks considerably. The Centers for Disease Control and Prevention (CDC) dubs the six highest threats as "Category A" agents. I call them the "Chessmen of Doom":

The Pawn: Botulism

The Rook: Tularemia

The Knights: Ebola (and other viral hemorrhagic fevers)

The Bishop: Plague

The King: Smallpox

And . . . the Queen: Anthrax.

Each pathogen has unique skills and attack strategies to outmaneuver humans and rain death and destruction on individuals or societies.

3

The Six "Chessmen of Doom"

Ring-a-round the rosies
A pocket full of posies
Ashes! Ashes!
We all fall down.

My job as chief of Medicine was to understand the microbial enemy. Each "chessman" has unique characteristics and capabilities to kill people. They have the rare virulence, shared by only a handful of diseases, to kill a healthy person within a week or so of illness onset. No wonder they scare people. Several of them are diseases of antiquity, notorious for wiping out countless humans throughout history.

It helps to know something about each microbial adversary's unique characteristics and their impact on history to avoid repeating it. The fear factor alone is contagious and can amplify the chaos created by the infectious agent and degrade a military's or a population's will to fight. If someone wants to scare people, why not reach for an agent whose name conjures up images of doom that anyone can relate to?

As in a fencing match, in the lab, or on the battlefield, we parried each one of the agents, as best we could, using our limited toolbox.

THE SIX "CHESSMEN OF DOOM"

The Pawn: Botulism

(Caused by toxins produced by *Clostridium botulinum* bacteria)

The pawn is the lowest of the pieces on the chessboard.[1] It moves one or two spaces at a time and can attack only from one space away. Similarly, botulism is the lowest of the deadly Chessmen. The causative organism was named after the Latin term *botulus,* "sausage," based on its elongated, cylindrical shape under the microscope and early outbreaks linked to sausages. Similar to the pawns or serfs from the Middle Ages who spent their lives tilling the soil, the bacteria that produce botulinum toxins live in the soil. They hibernate under hostile conditions in a protected seedlike spore stage. If you scoop up some dirt in your backyard, you might find some.

Botulism occurs rarely after home canning has gone awry because incompletely washed fruits or vegetables can harbor residual dirt containing the spores. Without adequate sterilization of the food before the can or jar is sealed, *Clostridium botulinum (C. botulinum),* an anaerobe, will proliferate without oxygen. Like pus inside a painful boil, *C. botulinum* festers inside the can while producing the toxin. We find out the hard way that victims have ingested the toxin—they die.

Botulinum toxins are the most potent neurotoxins on the planet—fifteen thousand times more toxic than the deadliest man-made nerve agent, called "vx," which North Korea allegedly used in 2017 to assassinate Kim Jong Nam, half-brother of the North Korean dictator. Just a tiny drop on the skin containing only 6–10 mg of vx is enough to kill a human. Botulinum toxins are one hundred thousand times more toxic than sarin (GB), which Syria launched against civilians. Only 1 nanogram of botulinum toxin (a billionth of a gram, 10^{-9} grams) per kilogram of body weight will kill a human. That's a microscopic amount, invisible to the human eye. The toxins kill in a horrific way, by paralyzing people.

The toxins' deadly features have attracted multiple superpowers. The United States sought to isolate and purify the toxin, calling it by the code name "agent X." The Soviets tested botulinum-filled weapons, and after the first Gulf War, Iraq admitted to producing and weaponizing it for missiles, bombs, and tank sprayers.[2]

Although deadly, like pawns on the chessboard, botulinum toxins do not have the lengthy downwind reach of the other Chessmen, so they have a more limited target range. They may be the lowest of the Chessmen, but sneaky "pawns" make good assassination weapons when placed in a target's food or on a sharp instrument. Some have speculated whether Reinhard Heydrich, Hitler's head of the Gestapo, was assassinated with a botulism-laden bomb.

Everyone loves milk—a staple of the American diet. Although botulinum toxins don't spray well over long distances, they work very effectively, and at very low concentrations in food. What would happen if a terrorist unleashed botulinum toxin in our milk supply? When I was at a botulism-preparedness meeting shortly after 9/11, Secretary of Health and Human Services Tommy Thompson, who sat next to me, told the group around the table that it was what he feared most. An attack could exact widespread damage across the United States, just as extensive as a salmonella outbreak, with over one hundred thousand victims—but with far deadlier consequences.[3]

The Rook: Tularemia

(Caused by the bacteria *Francisella tularensis*)

Under a microscope *Francisella tularensis*, described as a "coccobacillus," appears sometimes like a small sphere but occasionally slightly elongated. Tularemia gets its name from Tulare County, California, where it was discovered during a die off of infected ground squirrels in 1911. Among the high-threat agents, tularemia doesn't get the respect it deserves, and it is frequently overshadowed by its more widely recognized fellow Chessmen.

Tularemia causes similar damage as plague, but "only" kills about a third of its victims compared with plague's 60 percent or higher death rates, earning it the nickname "plague minor." However, similar to the rook (also known as the castle) on the chessboard, which can move in straight or lateral directions across the entire chessboard, tularemia has one of the longest reaches of the Chessmen. A release of 50 kilograms of tularemia upwind of a city of 500,000 people would strike >20 kilometers downwind, incapacitating 125,000 and killing 30,000 people.[4] Tularemia infects with very few organisms (~10) compared to plague (100 organisms) or anthrax (10,000 spores), one of the properties that make it an ideal bioweapon. Tularemia surfaces in large outbreaks, often during the breakdown of sanitation systems, so its name comes up frequently as a bioweapon suspect following the ravages of war. During World War II, Russian military and civilian populations suffered a devastating outbreak with over 100,000 victims.

The United States and the Soviet Union both developed tularemia as a weapon. The late Bill Patrick, chief of Product for the former U.S. bioweapons program, called it his "favorite" weapon because he could target the enemy effectively at different distances downwind.

....

The Knights: Viral Hemorrhagic Fevers

(Caused by Filoviruses (Ebola and Marburg) and Arenaviruses (Lassa, Junin, and Machupo).

Like the knights on the chessboard and their ability to surprise with a unique movement pattern (forward and laterally in the same move), the viral hemorrhagic fever "knights," like Ebola, are just as tricky in real life. They jump out from nowhere, decimate remote African hospitals and villages, and then disappear back into the jungle, not to be heard from again for months to years.

In 1967 Germany and Yugoslavia imported African green monkeys from Uganda for medical research. Soon thereafter, researchers who worked with the monkeys or tissues from them began to get sick, experiencing high fevers, vomiting, diarrhea, red eyes, and a rash. When the outbreak ended, thirty-one people had become sick and seven died of a new, mysterious illness. Two victims spread it to others.

When investigators viewed the perpetrator under an electron microscope, they discovered a new, bizarre-looking virus—long and spindly, like a snake or a shepherd's crook. They gave it a new family name to match: a "filovirus," from the Latin term *filum*, "thread." The virus itself was dubbed Marburg, after one outbreak site in Marburg, Germany. Marburg then went into hiding, striking the rare, unfortunate victim or two.

Fast forward to 1976. A new deadly outbreak with similar features emerges in the central African countries of Zaire and Sudan. Is Marburg back? The CDC launches a team to investigate. They discover not one but two new viruses, with the same spindly shape— close cousins but different from Marburg. Karl Johnson, the lead disease detective, names them "Ebola," after the Ebola River near the outbreak site in northern Zaire (now Democratic Republic of the

Congo). The two viruses become known as Ebola Zaire and Ebola Sudan after the countries where they occurred. The Zaire species appears deadlier, killing 80 percent or more of its victims, whereas the Sudan species kills "only" about 50 percent.

Why does Ebola cause such an uproar? Thousands of African children die every day from tuberculosis, malaria and other infectious diseases, but they don't make the headlines. The answer: Ebola is unique in many ways. Most other infections that kill so effectively have treatments or vaccines. Not Ebola.

Ebola is stealthy, launching intermittent, explosive ambushes. Between outbreaks Ebola hides in large African fruit bats living in the forest canopy. You wouldn't want to run into these ugly creatures with massive wingspans in a dark alley. Every now and then, a chance event causes a "spillover" into humans—when humans eat infected "bush meat" (small antelopes or monkeys), get bitten by a bat, eat fruit contaminated by bats, or have exposure to bat urine or guano. Unfortunately, we can't usually determine how that first human victim was infected because the person often dies before we can ask him or her.

Compared to many other infectious diseases, Ebola doesn't spread very efficiently. If someone with measles walks into a room, anyone not immune in the room will get sick. If an Ebola victim walks into a room, no big deal, unless someone gets up close and personal with their blood or body fluids.

What makes Ebola special is how it takes advantage of human behavior and the hospital environment to proliferate. When the first human gets sick, he or she does what anyone would do: seeks medical care. Hospitals or clinics in remote African villages don't have sophisticated diagnostic testing for Ebola or the gowns, gloves, or goggles needed to prevent spread in the hospital. Dozens of other infections in Africa cause high fever, vomiting, diarrhea, and body aches, so Ebola flies under the radar, while doctors consider the usual suspects, like malaria, typhoid, HIV, and tuberculosis. The hospital becomes the mixing chamber for silent, exponential spread, as the first patient infects other patients and the health-care providers. Then, wham, out of nowhere, multiple people "break" with Ebola fever. The knights strike down doctors, nurses, and laboratory staff, leaving the hospital a ghost town. Victims flee the hospital or stay home to die, and they infect their family members. Eventually, in remote areas without a fresh supply of victims, spread stops and the outbreak burns itself out. But what happens when Ebola doesn't burn out? Unfortunately, in 2014–16 we had a real-life lesson in West Africa, with over 28,000 victims and over 11,000 dead.

In 1995 the Japanese cult Aum Shinrikyo sent its members to Zaire during an outbreak to collect specimens of Ebola. The Soviets also sought to weaponize Marburg, but Ebola has not been used as a weapon. This has not prevented the media from fueling public fear, with books and movies like *The Hot Zone* and *Outbreak*. However, despite all the "sexy" Hollywood images of victims shaking with high fevers, bruised faces, and bleeding from their eyeballs, Ebola doesn't make a great bioweapon. It's hard to produce in large quantities, and it isn't very stable in the environment, so it would be hard to infect a lot of people by spraying it over a city or a battlefield.

Some of its fellow Chessmen may not scare the public as much as Ebola or Marburg or Lassa, but they make much more efficient germ weapons.

The Bishop: Plague

(Caused by the bacteria *Yersinia pestis*)

Plague is the highly respected "bishop," with enormous power and sway over the poor and downtrodden, through his links to rats, filth, and squalor. Similar to the bishop on the chessboard, which can move diagonally against an adversary along the entire length of the chessboard, plague can strike at anyone, including the kings and the paupers, even from a distance.

In 1346 Mongol invaders laid siege to the walled Crimean port city of Kaffa on the northern edge of the Black Sea. Stricken among their ranks with a devastating outbreak of bubonic plague, they decided to turn this affliction to their advantage by catapulting the plague-ridden corpses of their unfortunate comrades over the city's walls. Shortly thereafter the Genoese defenders inside the city succumbed to the deadly infection. As they fled the city, unknown to them, they ferried the microbial enemy on their ships back to Italy, germinating the seeds of infection for the Black Death scourge that decimated up to a third of the European population.

Some believe that the beloved nursery rhyme "Ring-around-the Rosie" refers to the Black Death. From this dark perspective, the words take on an ominous and sinister meaning:[5]

Ring-a-round the rosies—the red skin lesion caused by a flea bite

A pocket full of posies—a flower bouquet to ward off the stench of dead or dying flesh

Ashes! Ashes!—death, cremation of the bodies or burning of the houses? Some substitute "achoo" for ashes, signifying sneezing and illness.

We all fall down—we all die.

Under a microscope *Yersinia pestis*, the bacteria that causes plague, has colorful cylindrical rods that stain pink (Gram negative) or sky blue with a Wayson's stain, and with a curious feature, called "bipolar" staining. The ends of the rods stain better than the center, making them look, ironically, like safety pins—something we associate with protecting babies in diapers (before Pampers), not death.

We now know that plague spreads by fleas that feed on infected rodents, like rats, prairie dogs, or ground squirrels, so the outbreak inside Kaffa probably had nothing to do with the dead bodies launched over the walls. Instead, infected rats carrying the fleas probably traversed the city walls and spread the disease. The same thing happened when the Black Death spread through Europe and infected kings and paupers alike. Fleas seek blood meals from a warm-blooded host before they can lay eggs. When a flea bites an infected rodent, the plague bacteria block the flea's gut, so it feels like it's starving. It starts a feeding frenzy, hammering away like a woodpecker, regurgitating infectious organisms into the wound with every bite. When the rodent host dies, a flea launches like a heat-seeking missile in search of a new warm body and possibly an unlucky human target.

Once a person is bitten by an infected flea, the human body serves as a fertile growth medium for the plague bacteria to launch into explosive growth in the closest lymph nodes, transforming them into massive, engorged, and extremely painful "tumors of the groin" as described in the Bible.[6] The lymph node is now called a bubo, and the victim has "bubonic plague." Within hours the victim spikes a high fever and has shaking chills—the worst flu-like symptoms imaginable.

A victim can start out with bubonic plague, but some plague organisms break free into the bloodstream and land in the lungs, creating the deadliest form of plague: pneumonic plague. Fleas and rats no longer matter. Death can be spread, with every cough, by a family member, a coworker, a subway passenger, or even the family cat. Victims cough up thick, murky sputum that soon turns bloody as it eats away the lungs. These "bishops" can start a cascade that coagulates blood in cooler body parts. Fingers, nose, and toes turn as black as an Everest climber's frostbitten fingers. The Black Death has set in. Without urgent antibiotic treatment, just call the undertaker instead of a doctor.

During World War II, Japan's notorious Unit 731, a "research" unit, tested bioweapon agents, including plague, botulism, and smallpox on living prisoners of war. Under the leadership of General Shiro Ishii, they developed ceramic vessels to protect fleas during descent from an aircraft, which then dispersed the fleas after the vessels shattered on impact. In 1940–41 the Japanese were suspected of dropping plague-infected fleas on at least three Chinese cities, causing outbreaks where plague had not previously occurred.

Today plague can still inflict the same horror it did in the Middle Ages. Madagascar recently suffered from a devastating outbreak with over 2,000 suspected cases and 171 deaths, many from pneumonic plague.[7] Plague still stalks the United States, with five to ten victims each year, mostly in the desert southwestern states, where they have had contact with infected wildlife. Some victims die, despite the availability of effective antibiotics, because doctors don't recognize the disease quickly enough.

In 2002 a couple visiting New York City both came down with bubonic plague. The husband developed sepsis, kidney failure, and required dialysis and a ventilator. He survived, but stayed in the ICU for six weeks and lost both feet to the Black Death. His wife fared better.

Was it bioterrorism? No. Nevertheless, those victims set off a firestorm because the disease landed in an unusual place, New York.

It turns out the couple was vacationing from New Mexico, where plague occurs commonly, and the health department found infected fleas on their home property. That discovery might make someone want to relocate.

Plague has shown resilience over centuries to spread across the world. Be on the lookout for multiple victims coughing up blood. Plague might be spreading.

Finally, we come to the "king" and the "queen."

....

The King: Smallpox

(Caused by the virus *Variola major*)

Smallpox is like the syphilitic king inside the protected confines of the castle but spreading contagion to his concubines, who pass the gift to others. He wields enormous powers to fell the masses, by striking the match that starts the inferno that spreads exponentially from victim to victim.

Under an electron microscope, the variola virus, which causes smallpox, looks rather benign, like a brick or a pineapple, considering it has killed or maimed more people throughout history than any other infection. It spreads in multiple ways, directly to household members and friends, or through "fomites," inanimate objects contaminated by bodily secretions.

During the French and Indian War, British general Sir Jeffrey Amherst sought to take over the French-occupied areas in northeastern North America. He came upon the sinister idea of giving "gifts" of blankets and handkerchiefs used by smallpox victims to unsuspecting Native Americans sympathetic to the French. Around the same time that the items were distributed, smallpox outbreaks struck the local native tribes.

Ever wondered why Canada is not part of the United States? An outbreak of smallpox during the siege of Quebec tore through the Continental Army and contributed to its withdrawal. The British forces, inoculated with an early form of smallpox vaccine (called variolation), were immune, and victorious.

Smallpox virus lands and multiplies in the nose or the back of the throat before showering the bloodstream. Initially, victims don't feel anything, but the "king" travels to the spleen, lymph nodes, and bone marrow, where he continues to multiply. Around day twelve, the viremia (viruses in the bloodstream) explodes, seeding organs throughout the body, including the skin and the gastrointestinal and respiratory tracts. Now the victim feels horrible, with a high fever, headache, backache, and extreme fatigue. A couple of days later, the fever drops, and the patient may feel better—temporarily. Then the rash emerges—first on the face, the arms, and the legs, and then gradually moving to the trunk. Now the victim can spread the contagion to others. The extremely painful lesions feel like cigarette burns as they progress from tiny bumps, to larger, fluid-filled vesicles, to even larger pustules. Like coalescing water droplets, some pustules merge into massive, disfiguring pus pockets, transforming victims into "monsters" in a few days. About 30 percent of those infected will die. Survivors carry lifelong, deep facial scars as permanent reminders of the "king's" wrath.

Smallpox also spreads through the air. In 1972 an electrician who had traveled to Pakistan presented to the Meschede hospital in Germany with what doctors thought was typhoid fever. During his stay he coughed a lot but never left the room. A couple of days later, when the doctors realized he had smallpox, they hastily shipped him to a specialized smallpox hospital. They then vaccinated the entire staff and patients against smallpox. Too late. Very soon, eighteen patients up to two floors above the electrician's room came down with smallpox.

Baffled by how the contagion spread, investigators released smoke in his room and watched it sneak out the door, down the hallway, and up the stairwell to two floors above. It also flew out the window and up the side of the building. King Smallpox had covertly attacked patients along the smoke channels as they lay in their hospital beds.

The Meschede hospital outbreak provides a chilling example of how easily smallpox could spread, even when the population has received smallpox vaccine routinely. In 1980 the World Health Organization (WHO) declared smallpox eradicated. We no longer vaccinate people, so we are highly vulnerable to a potential terrorist who opens a Pandora's box and unleashes smallpox virus. Add modern air travel to facilitate the spread of contagion, and you have created a doomsday scenario.

Every head would bow before the "king."

....

The Queen: Anthrax

(Caused by the bacteria *Bacillus anthracis*)

We finally come to the "queen" of the biological weapons, anthrax. Like the queen in chess, she can strike in any direction on the chessboard and has devastated animals and humans throughout history. One of the ancient plagues of Egypt described in the Bible could have been anthrax: "So they took soot from a furnace and stood before Pharaoh. Moses tossed it into the air, and festering boils broke out on people and animals" (Exodus 9:9–10 NIV). That sounds like the scenario we all fear—an attack from the skies.

Bacillus anthracis, the bacteria that causes anthrax, grows in long, intertwining "boxcar" chains that look like tangled purple (Gram positive) hair under the microscope. Any terrorist could grow anthrax easily using standard agar plates infused with sheep blood.[8] Upon exposure to oxygen or harsh environments, the bacteria protect themselves by hiding inside a cocoon-like spore coat with onion-like layers to protect them for decades in the environment, which makes anthrax a great biological weapon. An enemy could produce tons of spores and store them for later use. In the 1940s the British arrayed sheep on a grid at successive distances downwind to test anthrax bombs on Gruinard Island, a remote island off the coast of Scotland. Over the next several days, one by one, the sheep stumbled and collapsed. Forty years later anthrax still lived in the soil, so the British had to decontaminate it before letting sheep back on the island to graze.

Queen Anthrax has the perfect size, approximately 2–5 micrometers, to fly past our body's defenses and infect the deep recesses of the lungs. She also spreads great distances: 50 kilograms of anthrax spores released upwind of a city of 500,000 could strike victims up to 140 kilometers downwind and kill 95,000 and incapacitate 125,000. It's no wonder that the Department of Defense (DoD) was hell bent on vaccinating U.S. troops against her before sending them into battle. Using a vaccine to knock out the "queen," the closest thing we have to the "perfect" biological weapon, makes a lot of sense.

As my USAMRIID colleague, Ted Cieslak, likes to say when he lectures on the subject (one time prompting a call from the Federal Bureau of Investigation [FBI]), "If I am a terrorist, my favorite weapon is anthrax."

4

Hoofbeats

On evenings and weekends, one of the USAMRIID physicians had call duty, usually to treat a lab worker with a vaccine reaction or agent exposure. We also answered the USAMRIID 888 hotline for anyone around the world calling about a biowarfare or bioterrorism crisis. Shortly after my arrival in 1998, we experienced a rash of phone calls for bioterrorism hoaxes around the United States, ranging from the serious to the absurd, although sometimes it was hard to tell the difference. A typical call might be about a suspicious powder found on an office carpet that turned out to be sugar. One evening in July 1999, while I attended the *Prairie Home Companion* show at the Wolf Trap outdoor theater in Virginia, I received a call from a police chief in the Midwest. I excused myself from the show and took the call seated on the grass outside the amphitheater. Someone had found an empty dog cage outside an apartment building and moved it inside the building's lobby. When the person noticed a note on the cage with the words "This Dog Has Ebola," he called 911. Emergency crews evacuated and cordoned off the entire building of about 150 apartments, hosed down the area with water, and then called me.

"What should we do with the cage?" they asked. "Just spray it down with bleach," I said, and everything would be fine. It took time to convince them there was nothing to worry about.

Unfortunately, I missed most of the show.

In the summer of 2001, the commander promoted me to chief of the Medical Division, where I would serve as his lead medical consultant. I accepted the position a bit nervously but embraced the opportunity to build my expertise and gain more leadership experience. I became accustomed to dealing with a new mini-crisis about once a week for things like immunization policy disputes, potential exposures in the lab, or personnel management. Most of these incidents were minor, like a series of tremors before the earthquake.

The big crisis loomed just over the horizon.

Most people remember where they were on September 11, 2001. I had just walked into our regulatory chief's office when her phone rang. Her husband was on the line and said an airplane had just flown into the World Trade Center. She immediately hung up the phone, and we rushed around the corner to the commander's office. There we watched the television, aghast as a second plane hit the Trade Center towers and burst into flames.

I rushed down to my office in the medical wing to alert my personnel in time to see TV footage of the Pentagon also in flames. Now, with the military targeted, we felt our own vulnerability. Could USAMRIID be the next target? We learned that the Centers for Disease Control (CDC) had evacuated. Shouldn't we evacuate too? Instead, Fort Detrick went to THREATCON DELTA: full lockdown. No one could get on or off the base. The military leaders had no idea what they were dealing with, so they wanted all available personnel within reach. The lockdown worked until the evening, when Fort Detrick's command realized they had no contingency plan to feed the entire base. We were then released.

By the end of September, things had quieted down significantly. Then, one morning in the first week of October, the USAMRIID commander cornered my fellow division chief, Scott Stanek, in his office.[1]

"Only three people in the building know this," the commander said before informing him about a case of inhalational anthrax in Florida. "Be prepared. You may get some calls."

Scott reviewed the call schedule to see who was around in case things got busy. That afternoon I found a report online about the same case and handed Scott a printout. Clearly, more people knew about it by then, but it appeared to be an isolated case. Scott took the printout up to the front office to show the commander.

The newspaper headlines were focused at this time on the United

States' push into Afghanistan and the attempt to rout the Taliban, with domestic concern for imminent terrorist attacks.

A couple of days later, I wasn't on call on Sunday, October 7, but as I sat in church with my wife and sons, my pager buzzed on my belt. The sermon was winding down, so I excused myself and left the pews to take the call from a land line in the church office. The page came from my colleague, John Ezzell, chief of USAMRIID's Special Pathogens Lab, and a PhD microbiologist from North Carolina. With his long white hair and full beard and sporting a black leather jacket atop his motorcycle, he could easily pass for Kenny Rogers's twin.[2] We had built rapport over time, and he frequently sought me out for medical questions.

"I need a doc on the phone with me," John said.

I dialed in and joined John and another USAMRIID microbiologist who were already part-way through a teleconference with the FBI about the Florida anthrax case. John's lab served as the FBI's main referral lab to analyze suspicious samples for biothreats. Several others were on the call, including the FBI's lead physician.

Robert Stevens, a sixty-three-year-old photo editor for the supermarket tabloid the *Sun*, had become ill in late September and was admitted five days earlier, on October 2, severely ill with shortness of breath and vomiting. He had died on October 5.

Although the FBI investigated the apartments where some of the 9/11 terrorists had stayed, tests for anthrax came up negative. Tommy Thompson, the secretary of HHS, referring to Mr. Stevens, had said, "It appears to be an isolated case."[3] Reports just a couple of days earlier had noted that "Federal officials say they believe the case arose from natural causes and not from an act of terrorism."[4]

As I listened to the discussion on the phone, I visualized the effects of anthrax on the body. Unlucky sheep, goats, or cattle ingest anthrax spores in the soil while grazing and get *gastrointestinal* anthrax. Human victims, like wool sorters, ranchers, and veterinarians working with large mammals usually get *cutaneous* anthrax from skin abrasions in the presence of the spores. In her quest for survival, Queen Anthrax made two toxins that gave cutaneous anthrax its characteristic features of a jet-black scab (or eschar) and massive surrounding swelling that were easy to recognize, making it treatable and rarely deadly.

The black eschar gives anthrax its name, derived from *anthrakis*, the Greek word for coal.

Inhalational anthrax, on the other hand, is usually a death sentence. Once inside the body, the spores break out of their "shell," reproduce, and manufacture a protein coat, as effective as chainmail armor, that thwarts the body's ability to fight the infection. The toxins act like a bomb going off inside a victim's chest, filling it with bloody lymphatic fluid, crowding out the lungs, and making it harder and harder to breathe. As the bacteria multiply, they shower the blood stream, like metastatic cancer cells. Wherever they "land," the bacteria reproduce and manufacture toxins that yield tiny explosions of swelling and death wherever they go. Within a few days, the victim succumbs as he suffocates, and his bloodstream fills with massive numbers of Queen Anthrax's offspring.

On the call I heard for the first time that Stevens's case was being assessed for public health as well as criminal concerns. No one knew how or where Stevens became infected. There was some discussion about the public health investigation into places he had visited, like Chimney Rock, North Carolina, where a cow had died and whether he might have been exposed to an aerosol from a stream near where he had camped.

The FBI planned to send their experts into the *Sun* newsroom to investigate and obtain additional environmental samples to test from Stevens's work area. They were still awaiting results from samples that the CDC had taken in the building two days earlier. The FBI called for advice on what protective gear their agents should don before entering the potentially contaminated building.

As I listened on the phone, the church service ended. The church officers came into the office and were busily counting the weekly offering. When I said the word *anthrax*, the room fell silent. The church officers stopped their counting and eyed me with alarm.

The FBI was also considering giving antibiotics to the hazardous material personnel entering the building to prevent infection. I recommended against that. It seemed like overkill because during the course of discussion, the FBI had decided to wear fully encapsulating level-A suits, similar to our BSL-4 lab space suits, but mobile and with their own self-contained breathing apparatus. Without a breach of the suit's protection, there is no direct physical contact with the microbe and no risk of infection, hence no need for antibiotics. My main concern was that, once started without any known exposures, when would they stop antibiotics? I had also dealt with enough adverse reactions to know that antibiotics are not benign. The FBI doc disagreed with me. Everyone entering the building would get antibiotics. What I didn't know at the time, and which was probably discussed before I got on the phone, was that some FBI and other response personnel had already entered the building without level-A suits, and those individuals could be at risk. Giving them antibiotics until the earlier sampling results came back, then, was reasonable.

Stevens's case was alarming. As I heard more about the situation, I wondered how his infection had really occurred. Infectious pathogens behave in certain characteristic ways or live in specific parts of the environment. Queen Anthrax is no different. Stevens had none of the risk factors usually linked to rare cases of inhalational anthrax: he didn't work in a wool mill, he didn't bang on animal skin drums imported from Africa, and he didn't work in an anthrax lab.

No. Something didn't fit.

I teach my students that any case of inhalational anthrax in humans should be considered bioterrorism *until proven otherwise* because it is hard to get naturally. It takes about eight thousand to ten thousand spores. In the 1950s wool mill workers were tested and found to inhale hundreds of spores routinely, but they rarely became ill. Therefore, it was unlikely that Stevens had inhaled the dosage needed from nature to make him sick while camping.

Anthrax spores don't just float around in the air. They need energy to stir them up to get them out of the soil and into the air. Even so most of the spores would normally clump together or bind to dirt particles, so they wouldn't have gotten down deep into Stevens's lungs. The spores would have had to be concentrated and in a form that Stevens could inhale. This has happened before, but rarely. In the old U.S. biowarfare program, inhalational anthrax caused two of the three accidental work-related fatalities from a bioweapon agent.[5]

Still in the church office when I hung up the phone, the assistant minister broke the deafening silence and asked me nervously,

"Doc, are we gonna be all right?" I didn't say anything but gave him the thumbs up sign and left, although I didn't feel completely reassured myself. The story still had too many loose ends.

Robert Stevens probably opened one of three suspicious letters sent a week after the fall of the World Trade Center, but the FBI never recovered the letter. The CDC had been alerted to his case on October 3 and landed in Florida the next day. USAMRIID launched three of its own scientists to assist. News of Stevens's death escalated through the Florida Health Department, the CDC, and the FBI.

On the same day as the FBI phone call, two other tests would come up positive: a nose swab on a fellow employee who handled the mail and a sample from Stevens's computer keyboard. Before the end of the day, the FBI would be placed in charge of the investigation. Over seven hundred employees at the American Media Building, where Mr. Stevens worked, would have their noses swabbed and tested for anthrax that week.

Sometimes it's easy to miss an outbreak early on until it bites us in the ass. Piecing together disparate clues to determine how and why people are getting infected requires curiosity, a healthy "index of suspicion" for something unusual, and sheer luck.

In medicine, there's a saying: "If you hear hoofbeats, think horses, not zebras." Common diseases occur commonly. However, on October 7, 2001, we had a stampede of zebras thundering toward us, but we didn't know it yet.

Two days after the phone call, someone put two more letters in the mail.

5

The Queen Strikes

On October 9, 2001, two days after the phone call with John Ezzell and the FBI, I was back into my normal daily routine of running the Medicine Division at USAMRIID. I had just returned from a meeting and found a yellow phone-message slip on my desk.

Mark,

Tom Brokaw called. Please call him back.

He is expecting your call.

I reread the note before it registered. Wait a second . . . *the* Tom Brokaw? *Shit*, I thought. *What could he want?*

My mind raced through recent events that he might be calling about but came up blank. Having Tom Brokaw call wasn't too unusual, I suppose, because USAMRIID attracted the news media like flies to honey. After all Diane Sawyer had interviewed our former USAMRIID commander, Colonel David Franz, about biowarfare, inside the Slammer, no less. Novelist Robin Cook spent a day with my Operational Medicine colleagues before publishing *Vector*, his medical thriller about anthrax. At the time Tom Brokaw was the anchor for the NBC *Nightly News* and one of the most powerful men in the media, so I admit to feeling a bit nervous about calling him, but I was curious to know why he had called. Before I picked up the phone, though, I wanted to ensure I had the right people in the room with me to handle his issue.

I grabbed the slip of paper and a note pad and marched down the hall toward the USAMRIID headquarters. On the way I ran into Art Anderson, an army pathologist with a soft voice and a relaxed manner. As head of our clinical laboratory and Institutional Review Board (IRB), Art's knowledge would be invaluable if Brokaw wanted to ask us a diagnostics-related question. I recruited Art to join me. Upon arrival in the headquarters, I also pulled in our operations officer (a veterinarian), along with the deputy commander, a virologist, for the call. The commander was away for the afternoon, so we huddled in his office around the conference phone on the large oval table.

Brokaw answered the phone himself with his unmistakable loud, authoritative voice and explained the situation. On September 25 one of his assistants at NBC, thirty-eight-year-old Erin O'Connor, had opened a suspicious envelope addressed to Brokaw with powder inside and threatening words about a biohazard in the enclosed letter. Some testing done by local law enforcement on the powder was negative for anthrax. Since then O'Connor had been having problems with a skin lesion on her left shoulder.

After a few minutes, Brokaw passed the phone off to O'Conner. She explained that three days after opening the letter, she had noted a sore on the front of her chest near her collarbone, like a mosquito bite. Over the weekend of the twenty-ninth, she became ill with a fever, and the skin lesion progressed to a black rash an inch and a half long "like something [had] gouged it out." She saw her primary care doc and then a tropical medicine specialist, who told her it looked like anthrax. She started taking the antibiotic ciprofloxacin on October 1. The lesion and fever had improved by this time, and she had a residual black scab.

The list of possible causes of a black scab is long, with culprits ranging from bacterial infections on the high threat list, like tularemia and plague, to more common viruses, mycobacteria (tuberculosis-like organisms), parasites, and rickettsia (e.g., typhus), but she had no risks for any of those uncommon agents. Although anthrax was possible, since the letter had tested negative that seemed less likely. So we raised the possibility of more common things, including an allergic skin reaction, a chemical irritant, or a spider bite, in addition to anthrax.

I asked O'Connor about potential exposures, including hobbies that could have led to the lesion—whether she gardened, had any recent insect bites, cuts, contact with fish, but making any conclusion based on a phone call is a challenge without seeing the lesion or the patient. Like buying a house without ever seeing it, there is usually a surprise, and it's rarely positive. We didn't have the convenience then of easily taking and texting photos.

A dermatologist was seeing O'Conner now and planned to take biopsies. He wanted to send us a specimen.[1] Although O'Conner had no ties to the military, Brokaw was very persuasive, so we agreed to accept a specimen to test. We told him how to send it to our Special Pathogens Lab, which linked in with the U.S. National Laboratory Response Network.

Art Anderson asked for the skin biopsy specimen to be shipped fresh on wet ice, so he could test it with different methods, including trying to grow anthrax. Instead, it arrived the next day bathed in the chemical formalin. This presented a challenge. Formalin is great for preserving tissue, but it would kill any live bacteria, so we couldn't grow anything. The other option would be to test with PCR (polymerase chain reaction), a method to amplify very tiny amounts of DNA to a level high enough for detection. Unfortunately, testing PCR on formalin-treated tissues was not routine, so the chief of our Diagnostics Division didn't want to use an unvalidated test and risk making the wrong call. Therefore, Art made thin slices of the skin tissue and stained them with routine stains and one designed specifically for anthrax. The special "immunohistochemistry" staining method for anthrax was developed by our own special pathogens chief, John Ezzell. It used antibodies to bind to certain proteins on the anthrax bacterial cell wall—like a key fitting in a lock. The antibodies are tied to a dye or something that fluoresces for easy identification under the microscope. As with any lab test, it wasn't foolproof. The antibodies did not necessarily bind *only* to anthrax. They could cross-react with other environmental bacteria—like having a skeleton key that unlocks a specific lock but also other, similar locks.

Art reviewed the samples under the microscope but didn't see any features of anthrax, even though the positive and negative controls he had used during the test performed well. Instead, it had the features of an allergic reaction or a spider bite. It was possible that he just didn't get the best piece of skin to test. A diagnostic test performs well only with a good patient sample. Anthrax dies very quickly once someone starts antibiotics, and O'Connor had been on antibiotics for about a week. The chance of finding intact bacteria in the wound at the time was like finding a needle in a haystack. Art's conclusion: negative for anthrax.

Brokaw had mentioned during the phone call that they also planned to send a biopsy specimen to the CDC, but they had not yet reached anyone. A couple of days later, the CDC made the diagnosis of cutaneous anthrax.

Because our sample was negative, Art worried that the CDC had jumped the gun. They had used the same test Art used. Art knew the CDC colleague who made the diagnosis, so they conferred, and he asked him to send the microscope slides for his review.

It turns out that, of the two biopsy sites from Erin O'Conner, the CDC had probably received the "better" sample closer to the edge of the infection site, which explained the differing results from our two institutions. I have looked at the biopsy specimens with Art, and I can see why making the diagnosis was difficult—there were some bacteria on the CDC sample, but they were very scarce and certainly didn't look like anthrax. The CDC team members made the correct diagnosis, but they made a difficult call based on a suboptimal specimen.

Lawrence Altman, a medical writer at the New York Times, noted that even the CDC director tried to hedge a bit on the diagnosis, telling New York mayor Rudy Giuliani that they made the anthrax diagnosis with "a high degree of probability." The mayor wanted something more definitive. "Is it anthrax or is it not?" [CDC director] Dr. Jeffrey Koplan responded, "Yes."[2]

A couple of days after the Brokaw phone call, Art showed me a photo of O'Connor's lesion that the New York City Department of Health had sent him. It showed a rough, narrow, black scab (eschar), probably two inches long by a half inch wide on her front left shoulder near her collar bone.

"Shit," I said when I saw it. "That's anthrax." I wished I could have seen it before, at the time of our phone call.

We didn't have the benefit of hindsight. The stampede of zebras had arrived. It was no longer a theoretical possibility: we were under attack. But at the time, we didn't know the extent or what was to come . . . that the criminal had mailed multiple anthrax-contaminated letters targeting media personnel and politicians.

The letter to Tom Brokaw that Erin O'Connor opened was postmarked September 18, seven days after 9/11, and mailed from Trenton, New Jersey—the same date and postmark of a letter sent to the *New York Post* and probably around the same time as the one to Robert Stevens at the American Media building in Florida. The letter contained a threatening message, handwritten and photocopied:

09–11–01

THIS IS NEXT

TAKE PENACILIN NOW

DEATH TO AMERICA

DEATH TO ISRAEL

ALLAH IS GREAT

By October 11 a third employee who opened mail at the American Media building in Florida tested positive. An intern who worked with O'Connor in New York developed anthrax skin lesions on her face, and a seven-month old boy who had visited a different headquarters for ABC News in New York the week before also developed a black skin lesion on his elbow. He was treated for a presumed spider bite until a blood test showed he had anthrax.

On October 13 the national news blew up when O'Connor's anthrax diagnosis was reported in the media. Anthrax was no longer isolated to Florida. Hundreds of New Yorkers sought medical care. The U.S. Postal service advised people not to open suspicious packages.

There was a national run on ciprofloxacin (Cipro), an antibiotic commonly used to treat anthrax. Calls to USAMRIID's hotline skyrocketed. Operational Medicine Division Chief Scott Stanek received a call from a man who asked, "What do I need to tell my doctor I have to make him give me Cipro?" Scott refused to answer, saying, "That's unethical."

Shortly before 9/11 the biodefense containment laboratory in Canada had conducted a research study testing how quickly spores like anthrax could spread from a room where a letter is opened.[3] The results were shocking: within forty-eight seconds, spores fled the room and crossed the hallway to an opposite room. Within ninety-six seconds they flew into rooms five doors down the hallway. No one could have predicted we were about to experience a real-life validation of the Canadian experiment at the seat of our government.

On October 15 a staff member in Senate majority leader Tom Daschle's sixth-floor office opened another letter and spilled the powder that was inside, contaminating offices and the ventilation system in the Hart Senate Office Building. Immediately concerned that the powder could be anthrax, the staff member notified the Capitol Hill police, who arrived minutes later. Unfortunately, they did not put on protective equipment until they were inside the office. Anthrax spores landed in the noses of all eighteen people on the same floor of the Daschle office, which included the first responders. The spores floated down one floor through a stairwell in the Daschle office, where seven more workers later also tested positive. Two others in the neighboring sixth floor office of Senator Russ Feingold also tested positive.[4]

The FBI brought the Daschle letter in a plastic bag to our Special Pathogens Lab for testing. Wearing scrubs and gloves, John Ezzell took the letter first to the BSL-2 Special Pathogens Lab and then into Bacteriology Suite 3 (B3), a Biosafety Level 3 (BSL-3) containment laboratory.[5] He slid the letter slowly out of the envelope inside a biosafety cabinet, his hands moving behind a pane of glass and a curtain of air designed to protect the handler. A fine powder wafted up off the letter, swirling in the air waves, like a genie escaping from a bottle.

John had worked in the laboratory for decades. He recognized immediately the danger of this substance, and it scared him. Afraid he might have inhaled some spores, he shoved the letter back in the envelope, hurriedly flushed his nostrils with bleach, because he feared he might have inhaled some spores, and left the lab in a panic. He hustled straight to our clinic looking for me. Scott Stanek saw him in the hall and recognized the worry on his face, different from his usual friendly demeanor. Denise Clizbe, a nurse who had a bird's-eye view of the main clinic corridor from her office next to the nurses' station, saw John rounding the corner into the clinic. She recalled,

"He was white as a sheet, and he looked like he'd seen a ghost. That was strange for him. He was usually pretty calm." I wasn't in the building when he showed up, so one of my docs treated him with antibiotics for possible exposure to anthrax. A few days later over lunch, he described to me the indelible image he saw in the swirling powder: "I saw the face of the Devil."

As the FBI's lead testing site, USAMRIID immediately ramped up to 24/7 operations, testing thousands of samples from points nationwide. USAMRIID's diagnostics team was quickly overwhelmed. Jeff Adamovicz, deputy chief of Bacteriology, who sports a long beard splashed with gray, reminiscent of Ulysses S. Grant, said things "quickly spun out of control because of the numbers of samples, advice on sampling, and determining what was and wasn't *Bacillus anthracis*." The army yanked anyone it could from other departments within USAMRIID or other institutes to assist. "They didn't have enough space for all these people, so they started working in bacteriology's Biosafety Level 3 lab," Jeff said. "I'd seen the chaos with the samples coming in—they were coming in the front door, they were coming in the back door, you had people literally bringing stuff in with paper bags, these sort of evidence bags inside, but they were full of holes . . . we gotta get control of this, and I'm afraid they're gonna contaminate the hallways."

Hank Heine, a Boy Scout leader and researcher in USAMRIID's Bacteriology Division, with a full graying beard, wire-framed glasses, and an outdoorsman's look, got a call from his division chief at 7:55 p.m. that evening to report to the division office. There the chief told him, "Well, you know what's going on today, you've seen the news . . . well the letter's here. You need to go back into [building] 1412, get some of that, grow it up, and you need to run all the antibiotic susceptibilities on it." Hank did as he was told. He needed to get the bacteria in the letter down to the individual spore level, which would grow into individual colonies of organisms that he could later test against antibiotics. Using standard microbiology methods, Hank spent the next seventy hours back in the lab growing anthrax from the letter and running the susceptibility tests.

Hank selected agar infused with sheep blood, which gives the agar a blood-red color, because anthrax likes to grow quickly on it. "The stuff was like baby powder," he said. As Hank inserted a thin plastic probe with a loop on the end into a plastic baggie containing the powdered spores from the Daschle letter, he was amazed to see the spores jump up and cling to the probe like metal filings to a magnet. Next, he dabbed the loop on an agar plate and streaked a line of spores across one quadrant of the circular red plate, like an artist drawing a brush across a canvas. Taking a new probe, he streaked through the original line and made another line. He repeated this several times, so that with each successive streak, the number of spores would be diluted down to individual colonies once the bacterial growth appeared later. Then he put the plates in an incubator and waited for the bacteria to grow.

Hank found himself suddenly in high demand, as calls came into his lab from others in the institute, our commanding general, and congressional offices. This was not surprising because what his tests showed would determine the best antibiotics to treat anyone with who had been exposed to the letters.

The next day, the Diagnostics Division chief called me up to his office. He was concerned about the high volume of incoming samples and the potential risk to his personnel from them, especially from the Daschle letter. We sat down at his desk, and he took out a personnel list and yellow highlighter. His hands shook as he drew the highlighter across the names of nineteen people working in the lab whom he was worried about.

I notified my medical team that we needed to get eyes on these workers urgently to evaluate their risk of exposure. We phoned each one, called them down to the clinic, and swabbed their noses to test for anthrax. We started eleven on antibiotics, but we urgently needed Hank's bacterial susceptibility results to know whether we had picked the right antibiotics. We also evaluated everyone's anthrax vaccine schedule and boosted some. The threat was real, so we couldn't be too careful.

When he had first received the letter sample for testing, Hank immediately dove in and thought "it had to be antibiotic resistant." Over the next day, as the usual shimmering gray/white colonies of anthrax bacteria grew and spread out across the surface of the red agar plates, he noticed that some of the colonies looked a little different. They had a less shiny appearance when he held the plate at an angle to the light. Given time the colonies took on a flatter, yellowish appearance, sometimes creating a halo clear zone around the colonies as they burst the sheep red blood cells that were mixed into the agar. Hank assumed the different colony morphologies ("morphs") to be bacterial contaminants.

On October 16 a bacteriology technician who was also culturing the Daschle letter samples in the neighboring lab, called him over. "Hank, take a look at this," she said. "What do you see?" Similar to Hank's specimens, some of the colonies on the plates looked different. "It looks like a bunch of contaminants," Hank said. "Well, they're all testing out to be *B. anthracis*," she replied.

So now it looked like the letter may have contained different anthrax bacterial strains causing the different morphologies. The technician sent photos of the "morphs" to Pat Worsham, who was the chief of the Genetics and Physiology Branch of the Bacteriology Division at the time. Pat has medium brown hair and blue eyes. Her reading glasses attached to a chain usually sit on the top of her head, which combined with her sandals give her the look of a librarian. Pat had published a paper on different colony morphologies made by "oligosporogenic strains" as part of her work developing weakened strains of *Bacillus anthracis* that might be used to produce anthrax vaccines. She recognized that the spores found in the anthrax letters were a mixed culture. "Logically," she said, "it would make sense that that might be some sort of signature," and that an "unusual mix of organisms might be useful." The significance of that finding would not be apparent for another two years, but it would lead to a breakthrough in the FBI's case.

On October 17 Hank dropped by my office to tell me the results of his susceptibility testing. The anthrax isolate had a "normal" pattern, susceptible to common antibiotics, including penicillin, doxycycline, clindamycin, and ciprofloxacin—similar to what would be expected from an anthrax organism found in nature. "That bug was a wimp," Hank quipped later. "That was a big relief on everybody's part," he reflected, "because at the time, at least we weren't dealing with something that had been genetically manipulated." I was definitely relieved to hear this because the standard antibiotics we had already used to treat our personnel, ciprofloxacin and doxycycline, would still be effective.

None of the nasal swab tests on our personnel came back positive. We later reduced the number of them on antibiotics based on additional risk assessment.

Unfortunately, just because something can be treated doesn't mean it is not dangerous. Additional investigation determined that the anthrax spores in the letters were the Ames strain—a very potent strain selected for testing possible vaccines because of its deadly properties. The Ames strain was isolated from a cow by a lab in Texas in 1981, but it was named after the town of Ames, Iowa, instead because when a USAMRIID scientist first received the strain from a U.S. Department of Agriculture (USDA) lab, he mistook its origin and named it based on the Iowa return address on the package it came in.

When Jeff Adamovicz, Bacteriology Division deputy chief, received another envelope for analysis inside a plastic ziplock baggie, he realized immediately how dangerous the substance inside the envelope was and that it had been engineered to be that way. "We were trying to work out a concentration of the spores," he said, "so we had to be able to get some of the spores out of there, get weights, and then figure out what the concentration was," but the spores were "so energetic that you couldn't even get them to settle in the baggie." He didn't want to open the baggie in the hood because he worried that the spores "would fly out of the bag" and his team could be exposed, even though they wore powered air purifying respirators (PAPRs) to protect their airways. He came up with the idea of trapping the spores in a corner of the baggie, heat sealing that corner, then injecting some water into the baggie so they could extract the spores safely.

On October 17 the FBI released pictures of the Brokaw and Daschle letters. Not surprisingly, based on USAMRIID's preliminary evaluations, the *New York Times* reported that the Daschle letter anthrax was "pure and highly refined, consisting of particles so tiny that they could spread through the air without detection." The letters contained billions of spores in approximately two grams in each letter and "could have been made by an expert capable of producing large amounts of it." The physician for the U.S. Capitol indicated that officials would "draw up the net as widely as possible and err on the conservative side and test and treat."[6] Eventually, 625 were identified for prolonged antibiotic prophylaxis.[7]

Next to our main clinic corridor, we had a parallel second corridor, called the "Project Ward," that we used as an inpatient ward for research. The entire ward could be sealed off as a BSL-3 hospital facility, and research volunteers lived there for up to two weeks for testing of vaccines made from live viruses or bacteria. This system ensured no risk to the community and the ability to monitor the research subjects closely for side effects. We had a full kitchen attached to the ward to feed the research participants.

John Ezzell confronted me in the Medical Division hallway with a highly irregular request. "I've got the FBI here in the kitchen," he said. "They want to test some letters in the oven." "Are you kidding me?" I was floored. "Very soon the American public will demand to know what to do with their mail," John said. "The FBI is trying to figure out what to tell them."

John had filled letters with spores of an environmental organism, *Bacillus globigii*, to be tested as a surrogate for the anthrax bacteria, *Bacillus anthracis*. He needed my permission to conduct a scientific experiment: to bake the letters at different temperatures and times in our commercial oven to find an appropriate setting that would kill anthrax spores without setting the letters on fire. The results of the experiment could be used to inform the American public how to decontaminate their mail safely. They had already determined that a microwave would ignite the envelope's glue. We have a saying in the military that "no good deed goes unpunished." Though I envisioned my military career ending—if something went wrong, I might get burned—I agreed because it was worth a shot if we could generate something useful for the country. I hoped that focusing on the greater benefit would be viewed favorably in hindsight.

Throughout this frightening anthrax scare, I was just as paranoid as the next person. My wife banished me to our garage to open our mail while I wore a mask. One night I awoke with horrible left-forehead sinus pain, worse than anything I had ever felt. The next

The Queen Strikes

morning I blew my nose, and pure blood came out. Anthrax causes local bleeding and swelling.

Did I get some anthrax spores up my nose? I wondered.

I'll never know. I resisted the urge to swab my own nose, but I felt some reassurance that if I had been exposed, I should have some protection from my prior anthrax vaccinations. But even knowing that did not completely put me at ease. Fortunately, the pain subsided over the next couple of days.

Sometimes, in the heat of the moment, while we are dealing with the routine daily work challenges, it is hard to recognize the significance of the events occurring in real time. When I received that first phone call at church from John Ezzell on October 7, 2001, and the Brokaw phone call two days later, none of us could have predicted we stood on the front lines of a national crisis that would challenge multiple levels of the government and the medical community. In retrospect Erin O'Connor's cutaneous anthrax case turned out to be one of the earliest identified during the 2001 anthrax attacks—a sentinel for the tragedy and the twenty-two total cases of anthrax that would occur, split evenly between cutaneous and inhalational cases. Five inhalational victims would die. We now know that the perpetrator mailed at least five contaminated letters on two occasions.[8] The initial wave included letters sent to the American Media building in Florida, NBC News, and the *New York Post*. The two sent on the day of our phone call with Tom Brokaw went to Senators Tom Daschle and Patrick Leahy.

The medical system is resilient, though. Eventually, as the news about the letters hit the airwaves, some anthrax cases were recognized, and some patients received lifesaving treatment in time to make a difference. Unfortunately, this familiar delay in recognition repeats itself with every new disease. We used to think of inhalational anthrax as a death sentence. We now know that if we recognize and treat it early, patients will survive. Six of the eleven inhalational cases survived.

The tragedy of the anthrax letters nationally and their long-standing impact on USAMRIID had just begun. We would remain in the national spotlight, for better or worse, for many years.

Years later Tom Brokaw testified before the Commission on the Prevention of WMD (Weapons of Mass Destruction) Proliferation and Terrorism that when he called experts at the army's biodefense lab, they told him that Erin O'Connor's lesion was a spider bite. I was disappointed to hear this, and it points to a fundamental misunderstanding of the limits of a phone conversation. All we could do on the phone with such a "curbside" consult was to render a quick opinion. We gave Brokaw a "differential diagnosis," a couple of *possibilities* based on the information he and O'Connor had given us: spider bite, anthrax, allergic reaction, and so on. Perhaps we weren't clear about that at the time, but we did take his concerns seriously, which is why we agreed to evaluate the biopsy specimen. Ideally, we should have been able to see the patient in person immediately after the call, where a full history, examination, and laboratory tests could have been done, but she was in New York and we were in Washington DC. Hindsight is always 20/20, especially in such a rapidly evolving situation.

Only six months into my tenure as the Medical Division chief, I was certainly getting the initiation in biodefense that I had asked for, but I didn't realize it would be so hard. Some days I would reflect on the simplicity of my earlier career, when all I had to do was take care of my patients. But I wouldn't trade the opportunity to be at the forefront of preventing further tragedy during nationally significant events. Queen Anthrax outmaneuvered us on this one at first, but that's why she is the "queen." Some quick action by a lot of people reduced the potential national impact, but Queen Anthrax would present challenges for us over and over in the years to come.

Just when I thought things would settle down from the anthrax attacks, I should have predicted that things were about to get worse.

6

The Nation's Bio-Emergency Hotline

The FBI and people like Tom Brokaw sought USAMRIID's help with the anthrax letters for a reason. As Willy Sutton might have said, "That's where the money is." USAMRIID's decades of biodefense experience and its specialized labs for containing highly hazardous pathogens made it the go-to place for the DoD and the nation during infectious disease crises, especially those related to biological weapons.

Over sixty years ago, leaders of the U.S. biological warfare program realized that they couldn't just make weapons; they needed countermeasures against them too. You can't make a weapon if your laboratory workers get sick. The late Bill Patrick, chief of New Product Development for the U.S. germ warfare program, told me that he could tell a weapon's effectiveness by how many people working on it got infected.

From 1943 to 1969, over four hundred laboratory workers at Fort Detrick became infected with the agents they worked on in the laboratory, with tularemia, brucellosis, and Q fever leading the pack. The infections drove the push for safety innovations.[1] So the army created the U.S. Army Medical Unit (USAMU) in 1956 for germ-warfare defense. Over decades, unit personnel developed and tested an array of diagnostics, treatments, and vaccines against biological weapons threats. They also established a lasting legacy of working on highly hazardous agents safely, as worker infections plummeted with advancing laboratory equipment, air-handling systems, use of vaccines, and understanding of how the agents spread. When President Nixon shut down the U.S. *offensive* weapons program in 1969, the *defensive* program continued with the establishment of an innovative new research laboratory at Fort Detrick: USAMRIID.

During my tenure as chief of the Division of Medicine at USAMRIID, I felt personally responsible for the safety of our laboratory workers. I wanted them to have the confidence that we would take care of them, as with any patient, without passing judgment on how they got infected during a laboratory accident. Preventing laboratory infections relies on multiple layers of protection, but nothing is foolproof.[2] We try to minimize laboratory hazards as much as feasible and train people to mitigate risks, but laboratory accidents will continue to occur, because just like with airline crashes, most laboratory exposures result from human error. Nonetheless, USAMRIID has an incredible safety record, with only a handful of worker infections over decades, despite the deadly pathogens that its staff work on daily.

Pathogens don't like to be contained. Their natural drive for survival requires them to infect in order to reproduce. So the government developed four "biosafety levels" based on the pathogens' ability to infect lab workers to thwart the pathogens from meeting their end game to reproduce. Like the multiple barriers we cross for airport entry from the parking lot to ultimately boarding the airplane, safety precautions and laboratory entry restrictions tighten with each successive safety level from Biosafety Level 1 (BSL-1) to BSL-4.

At BSL-1 there are no specific restrictions because the organisms used don't infect healthy people. Move up one level to BSL-2, where most hospital microbiology laboratories operate to work safely on familiar names like *Salmonella*, *Staphylococcus aureus*, hepatitis B, and HIV. Some of these pathogens can kill, but they don't deliberately fly off the petri dish to infect through the air. They require an energy source—a dropped vial, a puff of air, a cough or sneeze—to get them airborne or provide an entry opportunity through the skin, gastrointestinal tract, or genitourinary tract. As an extra precaution, though, we wear gloves and a lab coat, wash our hands, and work with the agents inside a laboratory biosafety cabinet (a "hood"), about the size of a refrigerator lying on its side. Protected by a glass face shield on the front of the hood, workers reach inside below the glass through an air curtain that provides an invisible barrier to rebuff any organisms trying to escape.

At BSL-3 we cross the barrier into "containment" because certain deadly pathogens, like tuberculosis, Q fever, plague, anthrax, and VEE, preferentially infect through the air—but we have a treatment or vaccine for most of them. The constant whoosh of moving air heard inside containment labs comes from massive air handlers that maintain a vacuum and frequent air exchanges to keep the pathogens from taking flight outside the lab. High efficiency particulate air (HEPA) filters "clean" the air of very tiny particles, even viruses, so nothing can escape. Waste must be autoclaved, treated with disinfectant, steam sterilized, or incinerated before leaving the lab.[3] Vaccines may be required or recommended prior to lab entry or work with a specific agent.

The animal rooms are the "wild west"—the most hazardous places inside containment but with insidious risk. Pathogens hijack the animals as hosts for replication and to help them spread when the animals cough up or excrete deadly organisms in their body fluids. Nonhuman primates (monkeys) can be especially vicious and take every opportunity to bite or scratch anyone venturing within an arm's length of their cages. I've had my own close calls. The animals launch their arms suddenly out through the smallest openings to grab the closest object, often unexpectedly.

The deadliest agents, like Ebola, Marburg, and Lassa viruses, are unforgiving, and we have no vaccines or treatments to block them, so we need BSL-4, "maximum containment." In BSL-4 we separate the person completely from the agent by confining the organism inside a "container" called a class III biosafety cabinet, or "glove box." As in the movie *The Andromeda Strain*, scientists place the organisms inside the box and then work through specialized gloves attached to the box, so they don't need to wear any other specialized protective equipment. This works well for smaller experiments but has less flexibility for larger animals or high-volume operations.

The second option is to put the scientist in a container, or "space suit"—basically a giant body condom—that receives pressurized air through a HEPA filter fed by hoses, similar to tire pumps, in the lab ceiling. Once connected to the air hoses, an air curtain sprays down across the face to protect the eyes, nose, and mouth, and air moves through a network of arteries to protect critical body sites such as the hands. If someone breaks a glove or tears the suit, the internal air pressure will spray any infectious pathogens away.

Calling the containers "space suits" is not too much of a stretch. Once the electron magnet engages and the stainless-steel door closes behind you, you are a captive without an easy, immediate exit. Your lifeline comes through air hoses, and you enter a private world cut off from the rest of the institute. You must trust your partner with your life, as you would a fellow astronaut. A slipup with a sharp instrument or an infected animal bite gives the pathogen the chance to replicate inside you as in the film *Alien*, with disastrous consequences for you and your partner, including an all-expenses-paid "vacation" locked up in the Slammer. It's no accident that it takes months of training for certification to enter BSL-4 independently.

Having such critical laboratory containment assets has put USAMRIID on speed dial for national crises, whether it's the White House, the FBI, the CDC, or the military calling. USAMRIID has shipped lifesaving botulinum antitoxins, provided vaccines to quell an outbreak of Rift Valley fever in Egypt, and diagnosed West Nile virus during the 1999 New York City outbreak. One USAMRIID senior scientist likes to say that USAMRIID is a "national insurance policy" against catastrophic infectious disease threats. One former commander called it the "nation's Bio-911," the emergency hotline to call for biohazard or bioweapon emergencies.

As the medicine chief, I found myself in the thick of many Bio-911 events, including some that came calling from the highest levels of the government.

7

The Pawn Comes Calling

On October 18, 2001, three days after John Ezzell's Daschle letter crisis, I was working on my home computer when my phone rang around 9:00 p.m.

"How many doses of botulinum antitoxin do we have?" USAM-RIID's deputy commander asked, his urgent tone of voice stirring a visceral unease that I used to feel in the hospital when a patient's condition was deteriorating rapidly.

What? I thought. We were still knee-deep in anthrax. *Now botulism?*

My division took care of a stockpile of special vaccines and treatments that the army had developed and kept for rare bioweapon infections that military personnel or our researchers might be exposed to. These included three unique antitoxins to treat botulism not available anywhere else.

I thumbed through my brown leather-bound day planner, its cover tattered from use, like a priest's well-worn Bible. As important to me as the presidential "football" with the nuclear codes, my planner contained everything I needed for quick reference: the on-call roster, key points of contact, treatments for threat agents, and entry requirements for each of the USAMRIID laboratory suites. I reviewed a spreadsheet inside that listed the contents of our massive walk-in freezers that we affectionately called "Little Alaska" and "Little Siberia." I told the deputy commander the latest numbers of antitoxin vials.

When I hung up the phone, I sensed that something ominous was in the offing.

Botulinum toxins—the "pawns" among the top feared germ

weapons—kill in a horrific way, paralyzing people from the head down while they are wide awake, something akin to being buried alive. Each toxin floats around in the blood in search of a nerve target. Our nerves communicate with one another, like a massive set of electrical circuits, but through chemical signals instead of wires and plugs. Like a ferryboat delivering cars, the chemicals carry a signal across a channel between nerves smaller than a human hair to stimulate nerves on the opposite side.

Once inside the nerve cell, botulinum toxins block the chemical release from the nerve terminal, paralyzing the muscles on the other side. Victims notice the blockade effects initially with blurred or double vision, then a dry mouth and difficulty swallowing. They become progressively more helpless as their speech fails, they choke, or their head droops. With larger doses the paralysis descends to the diaphragm muscles that control breathing. The victim suffocates.

As I thought about the horrors of botulism ("bot"), I picked up the phone to call one of my employees, Bev Fogtman, who kept track of our inventory.

Standing about five feet two inches, with wavy light brown hair, wire-framed glasses, and a tentative smile, Bev gives the government much more than she is paid. As the repository lead, she manages Little Alaska, Little Siberia, and many other refrigerators and freezers. When the refrigerators and freezers break down in the middle of the night, poor Bev fields a late-night call from the security guards—usually around 3:00 a.m. Then she schleps into the institute, puts on a heavy winter coat, and transfers everything from the broken freezer into a new one.

Fortunately, it wasn't too late in the evening when I called Bev and verified the latest numbers on my spreadsheet with what she had.

The phone remained quiet after that, so I decided to go to bed, in case I wouldn't get the chance later.

Around 2:30 in the morning, I stumbled out of bed and down the hall into my home office to answer the urgently ringing phone.

"I need you to pack and ship one hundred doses of antitoxin to Japan emergently," the deputy commander said.

Excuse me?! I was shocked. *Did I hear that correctly?* Most botulism clusters are small, with a few victims. *100 people? 100 doses? What the hell was going on?*

The deputy commander couldn't give me the full scoop over the phone—a matter of national security. At this point it didn't matter. I knew I had to drive back to the institute. I told him it wasn't just a matter of shipping the antitoxin. Our antitoxins were investigational products. They were not licensed. Mounds of paperwork would have to accompany the antitoxin, and someone would have to administer it. I needed to call in some folks.

I asked whether ventilators were available—a potential lifesaving measure for the most severely ill victims. The deputy commander said he would look into it.

The reason for my earlier feeling of visceral unease was confirmed by the time I hung up the phone. This was a disaster.

Someone must have attacked a large population, I thought. *But how? Where? Why? Had a terrorist unleashed this in Tokyo, the site of a prior nerve agent attack?*

If recognized and treated in time, antitoxin can halt the spread of paralysis but not reverse it. This is not as simple as it may seem because a victim presenting with slurred speech, drooping eyelids, or gagging may lead the physician to misdiagnose him or her as drunk, high on drugs, or mentally disturbed. The wrong treatment might follow. If the patient is discharged home, he or she could be dead by morning.

Like millions of tiny magnets, the botulinum antitoxins circulate in the blood, binding and neutralizing the toxins. The time window to treat someone is short, though, because the toxins enter the nerve cells quickly, and the antitoxins can't follow them inside. If not administered before the toxins enter the nerves, paralysis ensues.

We had to act quickly. With each passing hour, the numbers of victims could be mounting and their illness severity worsening.

I called Bev again and woke her up. I told her I needed her to come in to USAMRIID to help get a delivery ready, but I didn't tell her the destination or purpose.

My wife was still sleeping. All I could whisper to her before I rushed off was that I had to go back to the institute for an emergency. She was used to it and knew not to ask questions.

I threw on some clothes and stumbled down the stairs and out to my car. By then it was just after 3:00 a.m.

I held a three-way call with USAMRIID's deputy commander and commander during my thirty-mile drive up Interstate 270 to Fort Detrick. As we talked, my headlights penetrated the inky-black surroundings and shadowy trees as I left the streetlamps behind and drove north through lonely countryside.

We needed someone to hand-deliver the shipment to Japan and to administer the antitoxin.

At the time I was fighting a severe sinus infection and taking antibiotics. I wanted to go myself, but I shuddered at the thought of a sixteen-hour flight with blocked sinuses. The commander asked me who could go in my place. I had only a couple of other docs in my division with the knowledge and authorization to administer this type of experimental treatment while meeting all the safety requirements of the Food and Drug Administration (FDA). I first suggested Ellen Boudreau, my clinic chief. She had extensive experience giving experimental therapies. We collectively decided, though, that for something this big, a military officer-physician should go.

I had an air force colonel in my division named Carl Lindquist. Carl was an infectious disease doc on loan to USAMRIID for just a year, but he understood investigational products. Soft-spoken, tall, thin, with light brown hair, Carl was my choice. It would take a lot to stress him. Unfortunately, he had just returned that afternoon from a couple of weeks substituting as the infectious disease doc at the Landstuhl Regional Medical Center in Germany. Regardless, we all agreed that Carl was a good choice.

I called Carl at home around 3:30 a.m. I cringed as his wife's scratchy voice answered the phone, knowing I had awakened her. I heard muffled sounds of movement in the background, and then Carl's voice came on the line. I had awakened him as well. I briefed him on the situation. After some more muffled sounds as he and his wife conferred, he said, "Okay. I'll go." I told him to pack his flight bag, bring his passport, and wear his dog tags, and that I would be in touch later in the morning.

A single incandescent bulb cast an eerie aura over the guard station as I entered USAMRIID's back entrance and signed in with the night guard. USAMRIID was a ghost town at that hour. I passed by glowing red and green lights and the steady hum of the laboratory air handlers in the dark hallways en route to my office.

The austere cream-colored walls in my office seemed particularly stark at that hour. I sat down at my desk, pulled out a sheet of paper, and started to draft a list of supplies that Carl would need to administer the antitoxin: needles, syringes, intravenous fluids—anything I could think of.

Another colleague of mine, Dr. Judy Pace-Templeton, ran the Regulatory Affairs Division and had schooled me on the nuances of FDA regulations and investigational products. With medium height and mid-length brown hair that fit her no-nonsense attitude perfectly, Judy taught me how to protect my turf in the usual interdepartmental tugs of war when I was a spanking new division chief. We became trusted friends and allies as we supported each other through some of the battles.

On this occasion I realized that I needed Judy's expertise—and fast. Fortunately, she answered when I called her around 4:30 a.m. The deputy commander had alerted her earlier, and she was already on her way in.

When Judy joined me in my office, we sat on my beat-up white love seat and wracked our brains to finalize the supply list for Carl. Frustrated, I still didn't know the details of what we were dealing with and why. When I complained to Judy and described to her what I knew, her facial expression changed suddenly from concern to fear.

"My *God*," she gasped. "They've gotten the president!"

Oh shit, I thought. Suddenly, it all became clear. She had to be right. What else would have pulled us out of bed for these kinds of numbers? This was even worse than anything I could have imagined. Somehow, someone had "slimed" President Bush with bot. He could already be dying. It was up to us to save him.

At the time an Asia-Pacific Economic Cooperation (APEC) summit was being held in Shanghai. The president and his entourage were attending. That was the reason for shipping the antitoxin to Japan. Judy had put two and two together.

Giving an investigational antitoxin was no simple matter. You can't just line up a bunch of people and hook them up to an IV drip. You must explain what you are giving them, advise them of possible side effects, and have them read and sign a sixteen-plus-page consent form. This might not be so onerous for a research study without time pressure, but when people are scared to death from botulinum intoxication and choking on their own secretions as their paralysis progresses, it is hard to focus. They don't want to sift through a sixteen-page document; they just want to get an effective treatment and feel reassured that everything will be fine.

At least we already had FDA-approved protocols in place. Although each was the size of a small phone book, over fifty pages long, the protocol provided line-by-line instructions, like a cake recipe, on how to give the antitoxin. We took our supply list and multiplied it to meet the needs of one hundred patients.

Each dose of antitoxin takes hours to give in a hospital with an intravenous pump. That meant we needed a ton of specialized pumps. The deputy commander put me in touch with an air force flight nurse who was tasked with coming up with the needed supplies. I sent her the supply list and requested at least fifty intravenous pumps along with all the other equipment. When I talked to her on the phone, she was not happy.

"Where am I supposed to get fifty iMed pumps?" she asked.

"I don't know," I said, but I wanted to scream, *How the hell would I know? It's not my problem. Figure it out and get me what I need. I have enough things to worry about.*

We knew of seven types of botulinum toxin–producing bacteria: serotypes A, B, C1/C2, D, E, F, and G. Ordinarily, the CDC would provide antitoxins for botulism, but the CDC kept antitoxins on hand for only three serotypes, A, B, and E, because those serotypes caused the majority of natural disease in humans. The antitoxin must match the toxin to the letter for the treatment to be effective. Like fitting Cinderella's glass slipper to her foot only, not her stepsister's, the antitoxin won't work if you give the wrong one. Sugar water would have the same result. I had discussed potential options with the deputy commander on the phone, but Judy and I had to make a very difficult decision. We had three different antitoxins in USAMRIID's freezers. In 1990, while planning for the first Gulf War, the DoD worried that Saddam Hussein had developed a biological weapon arsenal, which included botulinum toxins. This was a problem because the enemy will most likely use the biological weapon that we haven't prepared for. Therefore, the DoD launched a program to develop antitoxins against all seven botulinum toxins.

Fort Detrick has a separate base known as Area B, or "the farm," a couple of miles away from the main base, where animals were used to make countermeasures or diagnostics. At one point USAMRIID housed horses there to make the botulinum antitoxins. Scientists injected tiny amounts of the seven toxins into a couple of horses over time—just enough to stimulate the horses to make antibodies against the toxins but not enough to make them ill. After all serotypes had been injected into a horse, blood was drawn, and the serum (and the antibodies in it) was separated from the blood cells to produce the antiserum/antitoxin. One horse, named First Flight, produced the early botulinum antitoxins. A memorial stone now rests in front of USAMRIID dedicated to him.

We wanted to select the best product to treat and protect the president and his entourage. One downside with the First Flight product was that the relative amounts of each antitoxin varied because the antibodies produced in one horse against the seven toxin components varied. It's like having a factory producing seven different widgets, but the workers spend different amounts of time making each widget. At the end of the day, they have produced different quantities of each widget. So a second product was developed to overcome that challenge. Only one toxin was injected into one horse. Each horse "factory" then produced a single antitoxin. The manufacturer then blended the individual antitoxins from multiple horses to make a combined product with uniform concentrations of all the different antitoxins.

The main problem with both products was their origin in horses, because they risked causing an anaphylactic reaction or serum sickness in people. The manufacturer removed part of the horse antibody to try to make the second product safer. Regardless, Carl would still have to give every patient a small test dose and watch for a reaction before giving the full treatment. Then he would have to monitor the patients very closely for several hours during the intravenous infusion. Normally, a single nurse would be dedicated to a single patient to give this type of treatment in an ICU. Monitoring one person was difficult. Monitoring one hundred people was impossible. Carl would have to enlist local assistance to help him once on the ground. The last thing we wanted was to treat someone for botulism, only to have the person die from an anaphylactic reaction.

We had a third product: Human Botulinum Immune Globulin (HBIG), made by drawing blood and separating the serum from volunteers who had previously received the botulinum toxoid vaccine. The human product had the advantages of a lower risk of allergic reactions and it was easier to administer—especially to large numbers of people—because it's derived from humans, not horses. However, there was one major downside: it only covered *five* of the bot serotypes, A through E, not all seven.

In the dark morning hours, Judy and I wrestled with the decision of which product to pack and ship. There was no perfect solution. Sitting in that lonely office in hushed silence, with the clock ticking on the wall toward our impending deadline, we felt the gravity of the situation weighing on us. If we made the wrong call, victims would receive the wrong treatment. Some might die—possibly even the president. We had no way to know which toxin may have been used as a weapon. We weighed all the factors we knew and took our best shot. We went with the human product.

By this time Bev Fogtman and her assistant had arrived. They tag-teamed counting all the vials and verifying the correct lot numbers. They packed up the antitoxin while Judy and I worked on the supply list and notified the army's regulatory person on call. Fortunately, Bev had years of experience packing special vaccines or treatments. She had shipped lifesaving bot antitoxin to Ohio for an infant dying of the rare type F botulism, when the standard antitoxins didn't work. She had also assisted on a prior shipment of Rift Valley fever vaccine to Saudi Arabia during a massive outbreak there.

Like building a small igloo, Bev chose the right balance of cold packs and insulation to maintain the cold temperature during shipment for a day or more. She had to figure in not only transit time but also other delays, like customs approvals. It would be a disaster to pack something incorrectly only to learn upon arrival twenty-four hours later that the product had thawed and was worthless. Bev lined the bottom of an insulated container with dry ice, then arrayed several layers of brick-sized blocks containing frozen liquid on top of the dry ice. Once she placed the antitoxin vials inside the container, she finished off with a few more layers of blocks and then a sponge to keep the cold in.

To ensure verification that the cold temperature had remained steady during shipment, the DoD used something called a Temp-Tale, a temperature sensor about the size of a small cell phone with a short wire tail, that was placed inside the storage container during shipment. When Bev pushes a red button on the TempTale's face to turn it on, a small screen displays several indicators. A sun shows the sensor is operating. The user can key in desired temperature ranges. When the package arrives at its destination, the recipient checks the display, which will show whether the temperature has remained in the desired cold range during shipment or whether it rose too high and the product may be at risk.

I eventually told Bev what was going on. She later acknowledged that her first thought was, *Oh shit.*

While Bev packed the product, her assistant busily printed and collated one hundred informed-consent documents for Carl to bring, which amounted to over 1,500 pages.

This all took a couple of hours. Then, when we neared completion, I received another call from the deputy commander: "Increase the shipment to 150 doses."

My God! What the hell was going on? Things were getting worse by the minute.

Off we scrambled to get more product, pack it up, print over 750 more pages of informed consent documents on our dangerously hot copy machine, expand the supply list, and package it all correctly. We worked tirelessly until the morning light peeked through my window, finally finishing around 6:30 a.m. We didn't have time to pat ourselves on the back. Carl's flight was scheduled to leave around 8:00 a.m.

We debated whether to use a police escort. Time was short, but we didn't want to attract attention. Around 6:45 a.m. I received the approval to do so. Fort Detrick provided a police escort to ferry me with the product seventy miles down the highway to Andrews Air Force base in Washington DC, where Carl would catch his flight. My house was just off the highway en route to Andrews, so I arranged to rendezvous with Carl at my house on the way. It was a good thing we had the escort. Without it we never would have made our appointed arrival time. We hit the usual morning DC gridlock, so the police officer turned on the lights and siren. I was amazed to watch the traffic part in front of us like the Red Sea for Moses. When we entered my neighborhood, I asked the officer to turn off the siren to avoid scaring my neighbors. I rushed inside my home for a moment and ran into my eight-year-old son, who was about to leave for school. He had seen me get out of the police vehicle.

"That's a police car," he said in a panicked voice. I reassured him that everything was okay and that I wasn't under arrest. I still couldn't share any more with my wife, who was equally concerned.

Our understanding was that a jet would be on the tarmac, being fueled and ready to carry Carl to Japan emergently. When we arrived at the Andrews gate, I assumed the skids had been greased, and we would be whisked through. Not so. Even though we were in a police SUV, we encountered a bit of a hassle. The gate guard finally let us through after we said our plane was fueling and we had an imminent departure.

We arrived at the airfield a little after 8:00 a.m. The next challenge was getting the product through the terminal security. The box loaded with the 150 vials of antitoxin was about three feet cubed—too large to fit through the X-ray scanner. The security guard wanted to open the box. I refused. I couldn't risk disrupting Bev's careful packaging.

I described in general terms what was inside: "A special medicine to treat a disease. I can't let you open it," I said. "If you do, you could destroy it."

After some more back and forth, the guard relented and called for a bomb-sniffing dog instead. The dog circled the package a couple of times, sniffed, and fortunately didn't get excited or sit down. The officer finally gave us the go-ahead to enter the terminal.

Scanning the multiple jets on the flight line, I couldn't tell which one might be Carl's. We were the only ones in the empty terminal. I paced a line in the white terminal floor while waiting, waiting, waiting over an hour wondering when he would launch—longer than I thought it should take.

Around 9:50 a.m. Carl's cell phone went off. He spoke briefly. When he hung up, he said, "Sec Def called it off."

What?! That was it? The Secretary of Defense called it off?!

In a matter of seconds, the long night's fiasco ended. Up to that point, I considered the possibility that this could have been a real event, a false alarm, or an exercise. Neither of us knew. We also didn't know how high up the chain of command this event reached, but now I knew: it had reached at least to the Secretary of Defense.

I didn't learn the full story until sometime later. This was not a drill.

There are numerous "sniffing devices" arrayed around important sites in Washington DC and strategic locations throughout the country. They suck in high volumes of air and concentrate it for automated tests for biological weapon agents. This sounds great in theory, but in a real-world setting, those devices have problems. The concentration of agent they detect may be higher than the amount needed to infect someone. So they might miss an attack, but people could still get sick. The other, more common problem is that they kick off needlessly for benign organisms that cross-react with the test for a threat agent, causing a "false positive" alarm. The tests are based on antibodies binding to targets on a specific agent. Using the skeleton key analogy again, the key might work in more than one lock.

Judy's hunch had been correct. One of the "sniffers" at the White House had detected a positive "hit" for botulinum toxin. There was a very real scare that the president and key staff members had been exposed to the toxin just before they left for the Asian summit. Our mission was to ferry the antitoxin to Japan or China to administer to the president's entourage.

While Judy and I had slogged through assembling the antitoxin shipment, unbeknown to us a USAMRIID diagnostics team had spent the night elsewhere in the building testing the suspicious sample to verify whether the "hit" from the sniffer for botulinum toxin was real.

The best test for bot is a "mouse bioassay." You line up a bunch of mice, inject them with the suspect sample, then wait. They will end up by morning either "feet up" (dead) with their backs on the bottom of the cage or "feet down" (alive) standing.

After the event I had lunch with the commander where he said that in the early morning hours, probably around the time I left Fort Detrick in the police SUV, he was awakened by a surprise phone call from Attorney General John Ashcroft. While on the phone, suddenly Tom Ridge, director of Homeland Security, piped in. Clearly, he was on a direct line to the White House. This was no minor incident. When he received the test results, the commander told Ashcroft and Ridge that the mice were "feet down." All clear. Once that information percolated through the different channels, the secretary of defense called off the operation. All this from a false positive sample.

As we discussed the operation later, Judy and I were upset. We had to make a judgment call on the best antitoxin to provide based on limited information. If we had known that our own diagnostics teams were simultaneously running the lab assays, we could have conferred directly with them about whether they suspected one toxin serotype versus another and then selected the product most likely to succeed. Using licensed, rather than investigational products, is so much simpler. Maybe the licensed antitoxin could have been obtained from the CDC, and thus we could have eliminated all the FDA paperwork.

Fortunately, everything ended well, but I shudder to think that the president might have died if we had picked the wrong antitoxin because we lacked a basic piece of information.

Condoleezza Rice describes this event in her memoirs and during an interview with George Stephanopoulos. "We were just a little unnerved," she said.[1]

President George W. Bush also writes in his memoir that while at the summit in China, on a video teleconference with a pale Vice President Cheney, the vice president said, "The chances are we've all been exposed." As the president notes, "At the time, the threats were urgent and real."[2]

That was the understatement of the century. Having just dealt with anthrax, dealing with bot was certainly feasible. What might be next?

Four years later, in September 2005, during a large antiwar protest on the Capital Mall, near all the major monuments, six automatic air detectors had a positive signal for the "rook," tularemia, another Chessman. The CDC wasn't notified for three days. The CDC then notified public health officials three additional days later. The Department of Homeland Security and the CDC took heat for the delayed notification. The sniffers appeared to work correctly, but the agent was probably something occurring naturally in the environment, possibly kicked up by the movement of the marchers, and not from terrorism.[3] Fortunately, no illnesses were identified.[4] Tularemia can cause severe pneumonia with only a few bacteria, so it is frightening to think what might have happened with such a delay for a real event and the thousands of people in the area at the time. We were fortunate.

The technology and procedures related to use of the sniffers have improved over the last decade, but like anything new, they have their limitations and potential pitfalls.

The botulinum toxin response was just one of many short fuse events that we dealt with in the aftermath of the 9/11 attacks. The following week I met in the White House with one of the physicians to discuss countermeasures. While I was there, he escorted me down into the nuclear fallout bunker underneath the East Wing to store some countermeasures. We walked down a carpeted stairwell, through the massive vault-like door. It was sobering to view the Emergency Operations center where the president and the National Security Council had met during the 9/11 attacks—only six weeks earlier. We went into the small medical room, filled out a log documenting the names and numbers of the medical products I had brought, signed the form, and set the products in the freezer.

This would be the first of several trips I would make to the White House. My Medical Division, our regulatory team, and USAMRIID's diagnostics team continued to serve a vital role in support of the national response after 9/11. We faced more challenges ahead.

8

Bioweapons 101

It was the perfect biological crime—almost. The year was 1978. A man stood waiting for a bus in London when someone jabbed the back of his thigh with an umbrella tip. Georgi Markov, a Bulgarian dissident, was known for broadcasting anti-Communist messages on BBC radio. The umbrella tip breached his initial line of defense, the skin. He felt immediate pain at the puncture site. Inside his body ricin toxin, delivered in a poison pellet by the umbrella's sophisticated, hidden air-injection mechanism, began killing him silently.

Although not one of the six top threat agents (Chessmen), ricin toxin is the perfect weapon for a Cold War spy. Easily made from inexpensive, accessible ingredients—castor beans—it is potent and lethal. Most doctors wouldn't think of it, so the cause of death would be missed. An injection of only half a milligram, just enough to fit on the head of a pin, could have been enough to kill Markov. There is no antidote. The toxin binds to cells, which invite this Trojan horse in. Once inside it blocks protein production, throwing a wrench into the cell's cogwheel, and overwhelming its repair mechanisms. The cells begin to die.

Death by ricin is agonizing. Cells near the injection site in Markov's leg would die first, causing severe pain. Local lymph nodes, the body's next line of defense, attempt, unsuccessfully, to block further invasion. Other cells throughout the body start to die. The small intestine lining disintegrates, leaving a raw, denuded surface that oozes blood into the bowel. Victims can bleed into their brain, heart, and chest.

Within five hours Markov felt weak. The next day he developed a fever, nausea, and vomiting. He sought care within thirty-six hours of the attack, but the swollen lymph nodes in his groin and the thigh lesion baffled his physicians. Within two days his pulse climbed to 160 beats per minute, and the bottom fell out of his blood pressure. On day three Markov's kidneys shut down, and he vomited blood. His heart's electrical conduction pathways short-circuited, and he died an agonizing death.[1]

Ten days before Markov's attack, another Bulgarian dissident, Vladimir Kostov, felt a jab in his lower back while walking in a Paris metro station. He also turned to see an attacker with an umbrella, but he only developed a fever. When he learned of Markov's death, he became suspicious and visited his doctor, who found buried in Kostov's back a tiny hollowed-out platinum-iridium ball the size of a ballpoint pen tip. It was filled with ricin. The assassination weapon, hidden inside an umbrella like something "Q" would develop for James Bond, was created by the Bulgarian Secret Service and the Soviet KGB. Spring-loaded and powered by a carbon dioxide canister, it injected the poison pellets coated with a waxy substance into the flesh of its victims. At body temperature the wax melted and released the toxin. Unlike Markov, Vladimir Kostov dodged the "bullet." The thicker tissue in his back may have kept the poisoned pellet from penetrating deep enough to fully melt the pellet's coating.

Biological weapons have a range of potential uses, from the individual assassination to the next level, targeting tens to hundreds of victims. We fear most the well-funded terrorist or the military adversary with access to the highest threat agents, like the six Chessmen, the ability to produce them in large quantities, and the intent to kill or incapacitate hundreds to thousands.

The Aum Shinrikyo, a doomsday cult in Japan, presents such a frightening worst-case scenario. Armed with millions of dollars, scientific personnel, and the intent to kill thousands, the cult was enamored of biological weapons. Its adherents first sprayed a cloud of anthrax slurry from the roof of an eight-story building in Tokyo. No one got sick. Next they tried to disperse the agent by driving through the city with trucks emitting anthrax through vents. Again, nothing. It turns out they had chosen the wrong anthrax strain: one developed to vaccinate cattle. After they made similar, unsuccessful, attempts with botulinum toxin, they shifted to chemical weapons. In 1994 they had a vendetta against some judges over a real-estate lawsuit in Matsumoto, Japan. They used the opportunity to test a homemade chemical weapon and released the nerve agent sarin on an apartment complex where the judges resided, killing seven and injuring over three hundred. After this successful attack, they sought a much larger target in 1995: Tokyo. Using plastic bags filled with liquid sarin, they poked holes in the bags with umbrellas. The agent spilled onto the floors of subways headed toward central Tokyo, killing twelve and injuring thousands.

Although the mistakes made by a well-funded organization like the Aum demonstrate that executing a large-scale bioweapon attack is not simple, it is not hard to understand the appeal of bioweapons. The incubation period of microbes (the delay between exposure and when victims become ill) allows the perpetrator to escape halfway around the world and sit on the beach nursing a gin and tonic before anyone knows what hit him. Some of the agents have vaccines, so the perpetrators can protect themselves. And with disease to cover their tracks, the perpetrators may throw off the scent of public health authorities who may assume the deaths and illnesses occurred naturally. It's hard to figure out when illnesses are not due to natural causes.

That's what happened in the Dalles, Oregon.

The Baghwan Shree Rajneesh, a spiritual leader with a long white beard and a penchant for Cadillacs, established a commune in 1981 on a ranch near the sparsely populated (<50) town of Antelope, Oregon. In the ensuing years, the "Rajneesh Purim" commune grew to over seven thousand members and developed escalating tensions and legal battles with its neighbors and the town.

Armed with a microbe weapon created by nature and using a laboratory on the compound, the commune's chief nurse grew *Salmonella typhimurium*—a cousin to the agent that causes typhoid fever. This was a strategic decision—to pick an agent that would cause severe diarrhea but not kill people. Typhoid fever kills. A rare and deadly agent like typhoid might raise too many alarm bells.

In a series of attacks in the fall of 1984, commune members secretly contaminated food and salad bars at ten restaurants in the local community. Then they sat back to watch the results: 751 people became sick with salmonella infection. Local public-health authorities recognized the outbreak and investigated. Some foodborne outbreaks can be linked to a sick employee. None could be found. When an outbreak occurs at multiple restaurants, the contaminated foods at each restaurant should be the same or come from a common supplier. They didn't.[2] The investigators knew the outbreak didn't match the normal pattern of a foodborne outbreak, but they couldn't pinpoint the cause.

A year later a cult member confessed to the crime, but what was the cult's motivation? The commune had hoped to keep nearby residents away from the ballot box to manipulate the local elections in a unique and sinister way—by making them sick. It was a tactical victory but a strategic defeat. The cult succeeded in making people sick, but it didn't win the election. An internal schism drove some leaders to flee the compound. The nurse who orchestrated the attack was arrested and jailed. The Baghwan fled the country, and the other members disbanded. Today, the compound serves as a religious summer camp.

Sometimes the terrorists aren't quite as sophisticated. In October 1996 someone brought donuts and pastries to share in the microbiology laboratory at a Texas hospital. A couple of days later, twelve out of forty-five lab staff came down with severe diarrhea, caused by *Shigella dysenteriae*, a bacterium that causes bloody diarrhea. When authorities investigated the outbreak, they linked it to the pastries, but they identified some odd aspects. They found no other local shigella outbreaks, so they couldn't blame the commercial pastry vendor. The strain of shigella that caused the outbreak was rare —with no cases in the community for years—but they found the microbial "smoking gun": a sample in the lab refrigerator that matched the strain isolated from the victims and the pastries exactly. There was no reason for that control strain to be out of the fridge, so accidental contamination from lab error was unlikely.

It helped that authorities caught one of the hospital lab workers, Dianne Thompson, on video bringing the pastries into the lab, which required a combination for entry known only to the lab workers. Oh, and she used her boss's account to email her coworkers, inviting them to enjoy the pastries.[3]

Using a strict definition, Dianne Thompson perpetrated a biocrime, rather than bioterrorism, because no one could identify a specific political, religious, or ideological motivation for her crime. We still don't know why she wanted to make her coworkers sick.

We can't peer into the mind of a terrorist. Sometimes the terrorist wants to gain a little publicity or just scare people. Whether it's leprosy, HIV, plague, or Ebola, infectious diseases frighten us, can create panic, make us want to run and hide, and can turn neighbor against neighbor.

It doesn't take much for a terrorist to prompt that natural, visceral fear of contagion. In April 1997 the B'nai B'rith mail room in Washington DC received a suspicious package leaking a red liquid. Inside was a petri dish with a threatening note, warning of the presence of anthrax and plague bacteria. Some employees complained of headaches, prompting fear of a chemical weapon attack in addition to bioterrorism. The security director called 911.

Within view of rolling CNN cameras, emergency response crews had approximately thirty employees strip to their underwear and hosed them down outside the building. The package was later deemed to be free of chemical and biological weapons, but that didn't matter. The damage had been done. The hyper-response was a terrorist's dream come true, making the national headlines, complete with the vivid video footage. Numerous similar hoaxes followed over the next several years after my arrival at USAMRIID, until local law enforcement and health departments learned how to handle them in a more measured fashion.

The six bioweapon Chessmen at the top of the threat list possess different qualities that a terrorist may find attractive. Only the "bishop" (plague) and King Smallpox spread easily from person to person through a cough or a sneeze. Ebola and other "knights" (viral hemorrhagic fevers) can spread too, but not without very close personal contact. All these transmissible agents can give the "gift" that keeps on giving. Once the infection is started, nature does the work for the terrorist, as one family member infects another, who then transmits it to a coworker, who coughs on someone at the mall, who spreads it on a plane, who brings the contagion home to another family on the other side of the world. The downside for the terrorists: they might catch the contagion they started, unless they have a way to protect themselves.

Some agents kill better than others. Ebola and Marburg sit atop the bioweapon "pyramid," killing up to 90 percent of victims in African outbreaks. We have no licensed countermeasures for either one. Plague and anthrax can kill just as efficiently, but if recognized early, we have effective antibiotics that can significantly improve victims' chances of survival. The death rate for botulism is highly variable, but like on a chessboard, a strike by the meager "pawn" can surprise. The first victims to become intoxicated (i.e., affected by the toxin) and paralyzed in a naturally occurring outbreak have the highest death rates because physicians may not immediately recognize the cause. Once diagnosed, though, quick treatment with the botulism antitoxin can limit the extent of the paralysis and save lives.

The human body has great protective shields against deadly pathogens. The skin provides a significant armor barrier. Our stomachs secrete acid to block entry into the digestive tract, and mucus and the cilia in our windpipes protect us against inhaling an organism. The problem is that these barriers can be breached or bypassed.

Organisms sprayed into the air may or may not infect us, depending on their size. This is a significant technical hurdle for "weaponizing" an agent: making it the ideal particle size to create an efficient killer. Anything below about one to two microns (10^{-6} micrometers) acts like a gas and floats in and out of our lungs without landing. Anything greater than about ten microns is too large to get into the deep recesses of the lungs. The mucus lining the air passages will capture the pathogen, and the cilia will push it out, like crew racers rhythmically beating their oars against the water. Eventually, the individual coughs up or swallows the invading pathogen. Particles between two and five microns are the deadliest because they can fly past the mucociliary blanket, land deep in the lungs, and start their deadly cascade.

Bioweapons don't do so well when released by an explosive device because living organisms die in the heat and light of the explosion. But that shouldn't provide any reassurance. Common crop dusters or other spray devices can be configured to release the particles in the "ideal" two- to five-micron range.

Some agents can infect farther downwind than others. If we had sufficient warning of a bioweapon attack, we could significantly reduce the number of ill and dead, but unlike bombs, chemical agents, or nuclear weapons, attacks with bioagents can occur covertly. We only find out sometime after the attack, when sick people seek out their doctors.

Some agents are harder to make than others. It's a lot easier to grow bacteria than viruses, like making beer, wine, or yogurt. Just swab some bacteria on a petri dish or squirt them into a nutrient soup. Add the right ingredients, some oxygen (or not, in the case of botulinum toxin), turn the incubator to the right temperature, and nature goes to town churning out instruments of death.

Viruses take a little more finesse. They can't grow by themselves, so they hijack a living cell to crank out their progeny—a much more temperamental process. Some viruses can also grow in chicken eggs. That's how the raw material for the flu vaccine is made every year.

Some agents are easier to obtain than others. You can scoop up some dirt outside your house to get *Clostridium botulinum* spores to make botulinum toxin, and you can find castor beans just about anywhere to make ricin. The multicolored, black-dotted beans are frequently used to make jewelry. It's a lot harder to get a sample of Ebola virus—you'd have to fly to sub-Saharan Africa during an outbreak and take some blood from a victim, or isolate it from a fruit bat flying around the forest canopy—not so easy. In fact no one has isolated Ebola from bats yet, even though we think it spreads between fruit bats when humans aren't spreading it. Plague or anthrax may be easier to obtain. You could look for anthrax spores in the soil, if you knew where cattle had died from anthrax along the old Chisholm Trail stretching from Texas to Kansas. Fleas spread plague among small rodents, prairie dogs, and ground squirrels in the four corner states of Colorado, Arizona, New Mexico, and Nevada. Catch some infected fleas, grind them up, and try to grow plague. The bacteria that causes tularemia also lives among small rodents or wild rabbits in several parts of the country, particularly Arkansas. Smallpox virus only lives in humans. Since its eradication from human populations, you won't find it in the natural setting anymore. It is kept locked behind multiple layers of security at the CDC in Atlanta and the Vektor Institute in Russia. Breaking in to get it would be an undertaking, like trying to steal the Crown Jewels or Tom Cruise stealing the "NOC" (nonofficial cover) list in *Mission Impossible*.

Chemical and biological agents are frequently lumped together as "weapons of mass destruction," but they have significant differences regarding how many people they can affect and how we defend against them. Mother Nature made bio agents. Humans dreamed up chemicals. They kill in different ways.

Although commonly called "gases" (i.e., mustard "gas" and nerve "gas"), many chemical warfare agents are really liquids. Sarin is approximately the consistency of water, whereas VX is more like corn syrup, but both nerve agents are volatile and evaporate. The vapors kill even if you don't get the liquid on you, hence the confusion with gases. That is why liquid sarin nerve agent spilled on the floor of the Tokyo subways killed people. If someone spills a chemical agent on the floor, it volatilizes quickly. By the time you smell the characteristic fruity odor of a nerve agent (Tabun, Soman) or the mustard or garlic odors of some of the blister agents, it may be too late.[4] You've been exposed. Bio agents don't get into the air that way. They need an energy source: a cough, a sneeze, a spray device, or a fan to make them airborne. If you spill them on the counter without such a source, they usually just sit there, harmless.

The other major difference is that your skin shields you against most bio agents, unless you give them an entry by scratching, cutting, or piercing it with an umbrella tip or other sharp object. Not so with chemical agents. They go through intact skin, like shit through a goose, straight into the bloodstream rapidly. That's why a mask and goggles may prevent exposures to bio agents, but chemical agents require heavy clothing lined with charcoal to absorb the chemicals and keep them away from your skin. Unfortunately, the protective gear for chemical agents makes you sweat like a pig. Soldiers are all too familiar with wearing this heavy "MOPP" gear (for mission oriented protective posture). Those scary-looking gas masks seen in World War I photos look that way for a reason. Chemical protection requires a fully encapsulating face shield along with specialized air canisters with extra layers to absorb the chemicals to protect the eyes, nose, and airways.

Because chemical agents are volatile, they don't spread very far downwind. Instead, once released, they evaporate into the atmosphere. When I teach about the differences between chem and bio, I show a picture of the Washington Monument, in Washington DC. Then I overlay the "footprint" from release of sarin nerve agent at the base of the monument. Like explosive devices, its impact zone stretches only a couple of city blocks. Compare that to anthrax, which can spread over the entire Washington DC metro area.

Understanding how the agents make us sick or how they might be used is only a small piece of defense. We need to exploit that knowledge to find ways to protect against them. As we saw with the Rajneesh salmonella attack, unfortunately we can't predict which agent a terrorist might choose, and we'll never have countermeasures for everything.

After 9/11 we had some experimental vaccines in the freezers for several of the agents, but we didn't have the luxury of time to develop new countermeasures. We needed to use the tools we had because war was approaching faster than I imagined.

9

Preparing for Biological Warfare

Long before September 11, 2001, we already had a licensed vaccine against anthrax to give to soldiers and lab workers *before* exposure. In 2000 the highest-ranking physician in the DoD wanted an additional way to vaccinate against anthrax *after* an attack on the battlefield, so this was a novel indication for the anthrax vaccine. It could only be done with an FDA-approved investigational new drug (IND) protocol and after documenting the informed consent of anyone who received the vaccine. This request rolled downhill to us at USAMRIID.

USAMRIID immediately put together a team led by one of our physicians who was an anthrax vaccine expert. After eighteen months and twenty-nine revisions, the protocol was ready to submit to the FDA for final approval in late 2001.

Then the anthrax letter attack struck.

This was no longer a paperwork exercise. In the heat of the anthrax crisis, the CDC, as the national public-health response authority, had no mechanism to vaccinate civilian victims after they had been exposed. Why not just give them antibiotics to prevent disease? That works for most people exposed, but unfortunately Queen Anthrax is sneaky. She hibernates inside lymph nodes in the chest, waiting for the chance to reemerge and strike weeks or months later, even in those previously treated with antibiotics.

We know about anthrax's method of hiding from monkey studies. One of USAMRIID's anthrax scientists exposed forty monkeys to anthrax spores and treated them afterward for thirty days with antibiotics. Monkeys survived while on treatment, but after the antibiotics were stopped, five monkeys still died of anthrax—even fifty-eight days after infection.[1] Another study from the 1950s showed living spores hiding in the chest ninety-eight days out from infection. Something triggers the spores to awaken, germinate, grow, reproduce, secrete their toxins, cause disease, and kill. Antibiotics may delay things, but once they are stopped, Queen Anthrax exploits the vulnerable window to exact her toll. In 1979 after an accidental release of anthrax from a biological weapon plant in the Soviet town of Sverdlovsk, some people became sick even forty-two days later.

Like playing Russian roulette, the revolver chamber spins, but we can't predict which unlucky victim will take the bullet. In USAMRI-ID's monkey study, only monkeys that received vaccine plus antibiotics all survived anthrax after the antibiotics were stopped. So it makes sense to give the vaccine along with antibiotics after an attack to those at highest risk. This gives them a fighting chance to build up a second line of defense with their immune system to knock out the awakening Queen Anthrax.

Because USAMRIID had already carried the new anthrax vaccine protocol all the way to the FDA, in the heat of the anthrax letter crisis, it was simple for USAMRIID, whose purview covered primarily the military, to hand it off to the CDC as a "boilerplate" for quick adaptation for civilians. Within days the CDC had a revised protocol and approval to give the vaccine as an IND to those at risk.

But after the 9/11 attacks, anthrax was not the only perceived threat. The new senior physician in the DoD, Dr. William Winkenwerder Jr., handed us another "tasker": develop protocols for the DoD's other unique bioweapons vaccines and treatments to be ready for military forces at war. The request split the threat agents into two tiers, with Tier 1 as the highest priority. Tier 1 seemed reasonable to me, focusing on three top threats: anthrax, smallpox, and botulinum toxins, but some of the products were not licensed and would require us to develop FDA-approved protocols.[2]

As the anthrax vaccine protocol experience showed, drafting any single protocol requires significant time and effort. Personnel in my Medical Division had practical experience giving one-of-a-kind vaccines against those threat agents to protect lab workers across the country, so we started a working group and plunged in feet first, along with our regulatory and virology colleagues. We held our first meeting on September 22, 2001—only eleven days after the 9/11 attacks.

I wanted the protocols to be nimble, easy to administer, and simple for a soldier to comprehend. I hoped to streamline them to two-page consent forms, with twenty-page protocols. In the heat of a battle or a bioweapon attack, no one can afford to get bogged down in paperwork.

I should have known better. After all the required regulatory language was added and after multiple levels of review, these documents ballooned to fifteen-plus-page consent forms and eighty-plus-page protocols. The botulinum antitoxin protocol grew to the size of a phone book, over two hundred pages long! It took nine months to launch our first protocol to the FDA, despite the urgency after 9/11.

We were now well into 2002. As we neared completion of the Tier 1 protocols, the White House started posturing for war with Iraq, so we felt pressured to get cracking on the Tier 2 protocols, which included vaccines against second-line threat agents: Q fever, tularemia, and three encephalitis viruses.[3]

Whoever had put together the Tier 2 list of vaccines had just looked on a menu of products in our stockpile and picked them, but the person clearly had no understanding of the diseases or the products. Although the idea of protecting the forces against these diseases had merit, many of the products were not appropriate for giving to soldiers en route to the battlefield. None were licensed. All were INDs.

Q fever and tularemia were already treatable with antibiotics. The Q fever vaccine required a skin test before giving the vaccine, or soldiers risked severe local reactions, so you couldn't just line people up and inject them all with the vaccine and forget about it. The tularemia vaccine was on temporary hold with the FDA awaiting new data from us. The VEE virus vaccine sidelined some people for a couple of days with fever, making them feel as if they had been run over by a truck. Around 5 percent felt as if they had the disease that the vaccine was supposed to prevent. The eastern and western equine encephalitis virus vaccines required multiple boosters. We really needed licensed vaccines, but none existed for the diseases in question.

This is nuts, I thought. I just couldn't envision vaccinating hundreds or thousands of military forces with any of these IND vaccines as they lined up to board and later jump out of airplanes. All recipients would have to be educated about the vaccines and their side effects and voluntarily accept the risk of getting them. Our working group decided to push back against Tier 2.

By this time I felt comfortable in my role as Medical Division chief, and I wasn't afraid to speak up. Our leaders at Fort Detrick listened.

So on April 17, 2002, I drove down to the Pentagon as the voice of the Contingency Protocol Working Group to bring our concerns to Dr. Winkenwerder and Dr. Anna Johnson-Winegar, the deputy assistant secretary of defense for chemical-biological defense.

I felt nervous. These were the highest-ranking DoD leaders I had ever briefed. All three military surgeons general reported to Dr. Winkenwerder, and Dr. Johnson-Winegar had significant power over USAMRIID. I would be representing USAMRIID on behalf of the USAMRIID commander and the commanding general at Fort Detrick, so I appreciated the confidence they had in me, and I didn't want to let them down. The commanding general would also attend the briefing, which ratcheted up the pressure.

We sat around Dr. Winkenwerder's conference table, with Dr. Winkenwerder at the head, Dr. Johnson-Winegar to his right, and me in the "briefing spot" to his left.

A colleague summarized the status of the Tier 1 protocols. I was up next.

We flipped through printed PowerPoint slides as I conveyed our concerns and the significant challenges of vaccinating large numbers of military personnel with the Tier 2 IND products. I felt pressured to rush, as I tried to explain the differences when working with investigational vaccines versus licensed ones, because Dr. Winkenwerder kept saying, "Got it," to move me along. I was concerned he didn't really get it, though.

At the end of the briefing, I emphasized that we still had the capability to vaccinate small military or special forces units, if needed, because we already had vaccine protocols ready for our lab workers or other "at risk" personnel.

When I finished talking, a hushed silence fell over the room as I waited for a response. Like a dog waiting to be kicked, I stared down at the last paper slide on the table, afraid to look up to read the feedback on the faces of others around me. I believed I had an equal chance of being applauded or thrown out of the room.

Dr. Johnson-Winegar broke the silence. "I agree," she said.

I could have hugged her!

After some more discussion between her, Dr. Winkenwerder, and my commanding general, Dr. Winkenwerder agreed with my recommendations. The Tier 2 vaccine protocols were pulled off the table. I felt a one-hundred-pound weight lift off my shoulders.

As I gathered my papers, I felt triumphant. I had helped stop a useless exercise, and at the same time protected my personnel and still offered an option to protect the soldiers at highest risk.

A couple of days later, our commanding general sent a note to confirm that the protocols were indeed off the table.

My elation was short-lived, though. By this time, I had gotten used to getting hit with a new disaster right when things started to go well. It seemed to go with the job.

I just didn't think it would come so soon . . . or from within.

10

Disaster from Within

One of my colleagues who ran a large research program once said that his daily mission was to "keep the wheels on the 'bus' from falling off while driving ninety miles an hour down the highway." On many days as a division chief, I felt the same way—like I held my finger in the dyke just long enough for another place to spring a leak.

I didn't have time to gloat over my recent success because one day after the Winkenwerder brief, another crisis developed. On a Thursday afternoon, April 18, 2002, around 5:00 p.m., the acting institute commander, stepped into my office and closed the door.

"How's it going?" the colonel said.

My suspicion meter jumped immediately because he rarely walked down to my wing of the building. Something was up, and it probably wasn't good.

Dressed in his army green "class B" uniform with wire-frame glasses accenting his square face, the colonel had something of an academic air. He sat down on the beat-up white love seat next to my desk and tried to make small talk.

I decided to make it easier for him to get to the point. "So what's going on?" I asked.

My instincts were spot on. The colonel leaned forward on the edge of the love seat. As he described the situation, I felt the white cinder block walls in my office closing in. The more I heard, the more claustrophobic I felt.

Although we were only seven months out from 9/11 and the anthrax letter attacks, the institute still ran high-volume operations in the Special Pathogens Lab, testing thousands of samples from the FBI for anthrax. The lab work was conducted in the BSL-3 lab suite called B3. Because of the high-op tempo, work had spilled out to other parts of the institute. One of the Bacteriology Division scientists became concerned about potential anthrax contamination in his office because some lab colleagues had borrowed his desk and left the area a mess. Dr. Bruce Ivins, one of the nation's leading experts on anthrax, took swab samples around his office for anthrax testing. This was highly irregular without first informing a supervisor, but his paranoia was apparently not unfounded: BINGO. Some of the samples came up "hot" (positive) for anthrax spores.

The colonel didn't know the extent of contamination yet. A lab team had been assembled rapidly and planned to work through the night collecting and testing samples taken from throughout the institute to verify whether the positive samples thus far were the real thing and not some other harmless organism.

"I wanted to give you a heads up to start planning your response in case more samples come up hot," the colonel told me. "Thanks, I appreciate it," I said. "Keep it 'close hold' for now," he advised, with the exception that I could confer with other doctors in my division.

Before leaving, he requested my presence at a meeting of the key decision makers at eight o'clock the next morning in the headquarters, when we would review the results from the overnight sampling and come up with a plan.

"Wonderful," I said sarcastically. "I can't wait."

"Another chance to excel!" the colonel said flippantly as he left my office.

I had a significantly different opinion. There was no way to sugarcoat this. It was a freaking disaster! I started asking myself key questions and running scenarios as my mind went into overdrive. Where else was the contamination? Who was at risk? What kind of risk did they face? How can we determine that? Was anyone already sick? Who should receive antibiotics? Do I need to treat all six hundred employees or a targeted group? Who else needs to know?

Most people had already left for the day. I didn't think I knew enough yet to alarm my fellow Division of Medicine physicians, but I immediately hustled down the hall to Scott Stanek's office. Scott, who owned the Slammer space, ran the Operational Medicine Division and was a seasoned public health physician with an even keel and a quiet, thoughtful demeanor. He frequently served as my sounding board, and vice versa, because I trusted his opinion. Scott also had several physicians working for him who could back my team up if a stampede of panicked employees overwhelmed us.

I brought Scott up to speed, and we discussed the potential implications. He agreed with me. It was too early to make any decisions until we had more information from the overnight sampling, but we needed to prepare to spin up operations quickly.

That night at home, as usual, I didn't tell my wife about this latest crisis. I preferred to keep similar issues to myself until they became public. My natural tendency is to internalize stress, while trying to project an external calm demeanor. Consequently, the tension burns in my gut like a bed of hot embers. I tossed and turned the whole night wrestling with several "worst case" scenarios and how to respond. At a minimum some workers in the Bacteriology Division could be at risk, but my biggest fear was that spores had gone airborne through the ventilation system. That could put everyone in the institute at risk, and I might have to give antibiotics to over six hundred workers. Even if only a few employees were exposed, we might have to give antibiotics to many more because we couldn't risk missing anyone. The health and safety of everyone in the institute was on the line, and possibly by extension any family members through contaminated clothing or shoes, although that was much less likely. It might be hard to prove a lack of risk, though.

This could be a huge public relations disaster—one more opportunity to make the front-page headlines of the *Washington Post*. Containment labs have earned that designation for a reason—they are supposed to *contain* the pathogens. Agents aren't supposed to break out of the lab, like Clint Eastwood in *Escape from Alcatraz*. I wondered, "How did this escape?" and I walked through the possibilities in my head.

Researchers enter the BSL-3 lab through the "cold" side locker room, where they shed their street clothes and don scrubs. Then they move through a passageway to cross over to the "hot" side. The direction of the airflow moves from the exterior hallway down the main suite corridor and into individual labs. Upon exiting, researchers remove their scrubs and "shower out" before returning to the locker room.

Pathogens have only a couple of ways to escape the containment laboratory. Someone could sneak them out deliberately, but he or she would need to hide them, possibly where the "sun don't shine," while stripped naked and showering out. A pathogen could hitch a ride on the person's skin or in his or her hair, if the person didn't wash up thoroughly. If he or she became infected in the lab, once ill, the person might infect others outside the lab.

Airlocks are used to move large equipment in or out of each containment suite. If the standard decontamination procedure failed, a pathogen could stow away on contaminated equipment.

Each suite of labs has a "dunk tank," about the size of a two-drawer filing cabinet, filled with a decontamination solution. It sits in the laboratory wall with openings inside and outside the lab that are separated by a central baffle. If someone wants to "dunk out" a sample to outside the lab, he or she seals it inside two layers of plastic, decontaminates the outer surface, and then submerges it in the solution under the baffle. Someone in the hallway outside the lab then accesses the dunk tank and takes the sample elsewhere for testing or for storage.

Each lab suite also has a "pass-box" about the size of a breadbox, embedded and sealed into the lab walls, with openings on both sides, for moving small objects, such as lab notebooks or individual papers, in or out of the laboratory safely. An ultraviolet (uv) light inside the box turns on to kill any live organisms.

I welcomed the next morning's sunrise and an end to my torture of uncertainty. At least I hoped to learn enough details to develop an action plan after the morning's meeting.

When I arrived at my office, I noticed a small, red, circular sticky tab on my doorknob with a number on it. Someone had swabbed my door overnight to test for anthrax. It was a sobering moment. Prior to this I had not considered my own risk of exposure and illness.

As I made my way to the headquarters for the 8:00 a.m. meeting, I noticed numerous similar numbered tabs attached to door handles, walls, machinery, and other locations along the hallways.

By this time I had become all too familiar with the commander's office in the headquarters. His large oval conference table that seated twelve or so people dominated the room. A map of the world, symbolic of USAMRIID's global reach, covered the center of the table and was protected by a large glass plate. Several covers from medical journals showing colorful photographs of pathogens taken by USAMRIID scientists were arrayed at the head of the table where the commander usually sat.

I joined about ten of the senior institute leaders around the conference table. The commander phoned in from Chicago, where he was lecturing, and our commanding general's chief of staff dialed in from his office on the other side of Fort Detrick.

The deputy commander rolled out a large floor plan of the institute on the table, and he pointed out the locations of the sample testing conducted overnight, and the positive and negative results known thus far. We didn't have all the results yet, but the team had taken over eight hundred swab samples throughout the institute on April 18 and 19.

As I heard the testing results, I felt relieved to learn that the contamination appeared to be more confined than I had anticipated. Only three locations came up hot for anthrax. The bulk of contamination was centered around the B3 lab pass-box, with over two hundred spores, so that appeared to be a potential source for the spores escaping the lab. Bruce's office and the B3 locker room had only three or fewer colonies of anthrax. None of the other sampling sites in the building came up hot.

Even if some spores had gotten into the air around the pass-box, the directional air flow in that area of the building would confine their spread and clear them from the air quickly. A large airborne breach was unlikely.

The meeting lasted about an hour, at which time the acting commander announced that he would hold a town hall meeting with the entire institute in the main auditorium—at 10:00 a.m. The featured speakers would include himself, the deputy commander; the chief of Safety; and Lieutenant Colonel Kortepeter, chief of Medicine.

What?! I almost coughed up my breakfast! I had only forty minutes to prepare something intelligent to reassure the entire institute.

Having dealt with other volatile issues before, I knew that employees with any concern would come see us in the Medical Division clinic. So I had to prepare my division personnel— and fast. My mind raced to come up with solutions as I rushed back to the medical ward and called my medical staff together.[1] I wanted to ensure that they agreed with my risk assessment that we had a focused area of contamination and, therefore, a limited number of employees at risk. The entire institute did not need to take antibiotics. However, to prepare for a likely deluge of worried workers, we would cancel the usual clinic activities. All agreed with my assessment.

After we met, I had only a couple of minutes left to organize my thoughts. I jotted down some key messages and bullet points on a yellow legal pad, then headed to the auditorium.

Over the course of two town hall meetings, the entire institute of over six hundred workers packed into our main auditorium with standing room only. The acting commander spoke first, followed by the deputy commander, who reviewed what had happened. The chief of Safety came up next and stated that there was no recognized breach of laboratory safety. I was next.

I took a deep breath and approached the podium.

"As chief of the Medical Division," I said, while trying to steady my voice and hide my shaking legs, "the safety of the workforce is my highest priority. I believe the risk to personnel from the contamination to be low for several reasons: we have not had any reports of illness among the workforce; the contamination appears to be localized in a remote hallway that few people enter; if there had been any aerosolization of spores, the directional airflow in the building would reduce any risk of exposures; and most of the people who work in or near the contaminated area would have been vaccinated already against anthrax."

We had no way of knowing how long the contamination had been there, but as far as we could tell at the time, no one had been infected thus far. We had that in our favor.

As I concluded, I said "We specifically want to see anyone who worked in the contaminated hallway or who worked in suite B3, but any other concerned individuals should feel free to come see us." Anyone could make an appointment, and we would start seeing workers at 1:00 p.m.

When the town hall meetings ended, I was pleased that the workforce seemed reassured, and I didn't hear any grumblings. When I returned to my office, I asked my chief nurse to draft a one-page assessment form that we could place in a worker's medical record that would document (1) where the person worked; (2) whether he or she had entered the contaminated hallway; (3) whether the person had received anthrax vaccination; and (4) whether he or she had been ill. This would help us divide those with bona fide risk from the worried well.

At 1:00 p.m., as a flood of workers arrived in our clinic, we learned quickly the limits of our risk communication. Many workers were confused about which section of the building had come up hot, but once we showed them the building floor plan, we alleviated a lot of fear. Some weren't too worried for themselves, but family members had nagged them to get checked. Many just wanted us to swab their noses to test for anthrax for their peace of mind—just to be sure.

News travels fast around the Washington DC Beltway. The command realized that shortly before we discovered the contamination, an entourage of Senate staffers had visited the institute for a "dog and pony show" and tour. Not surprisingly, once they learned about the contamination, the staffers were upset and called to ask about their risk. The deputy commander called me up to the headquarters around 3:30 p.m. on Friday and gave me another "opportunity to excel."

He told me to drive down to Washington DC to brief the senator and explain the situation. He pulled out a map of the institute and drew on it the exact route the group had taken during their tour and the locations of contamination, so I could show the senator. I asked if I could bring Scott Stanek as my "wing man" and to take notes, because I knew I would be an easy punching bag. The deputy commander refused, so I went alone. Before leaving I touched base with the senator's medical advisor, a navy commander, then I rushed off on a fifty-mile drive south on Interstate 270 toward Washington. On the way I repeated nervously my upcoming dialogue of reassurance for the senator and her staff.

I crossed the Arlington Bridge into DC around 4:30 p.m. and slammed into a wall of traffic. A running competition had concluded around that time near the Capitol Mall. It took me an hour to move one block. As the clock ticked toward the end of the workday, I had repeated conversations on my cell phone with the senator's medical advisor. After sitting in traffic for over an hour, she finally told me she had brought the senator up to speed, everyone was reassured, and I was off the hook. Even though it all felt like a wild goose chase, I breathed a sigh of relief and gradually crept my way back out of DC.

From Friday afternoon through Saturday, we saw eighty-eight workers and took fifty-seven nasal swabs for anthrax. We placed nine on antibiotic prophylaxis with doxycycline initially (ciprofloxacin had been depleted across the country), but we discontinued it after seventy-two hours because we reassessed the risk to be low. All swab tests came back negative for anthrax.

The institute put out a press release. The army has an adage that "bad news doesn't improve with age." If we hadn't made the incident public, someone would have leaked it anyway.

The national news reports varied in their support and criticism. In one article a sympathetic CDC colleague noted, "If it can happen to USAMRIID, it can happen to anyone." An academic anthrax expert had a different view, saying the event was "highly embarrassing," and "evidence of a lack of leadership."[2]

Despite the negative press, at this point, things were looking up. We had not seen any illness among the workforce, and we had managed the onslaught of concerned workers. Unfortunately, almost on cue something jumped up and bit us in the ass. The institute contracted with a company for laundry services that employed handicapped individuals. We had inadvertently left the laundry company out of the information chain. Because we found contamination in the B3 lab locker room, it was conceivable that some spores might have hitched a ride out of the building on contaminated laundry. Regardless how unlikely this might be, we had to jump on it.

As soon as he returned from Chicago, the USAMRIID commander held a meeting early Saturday morning for an update with the key institute leaders as well as our commanding general. Things were generally under control, although we were just beginning to deal with the laundry situation. The general pulled in a team from the army's environmental center to test the laundry facility for anthrax.

During the meeting I happened to look out the window and was surprised to see an unexpected visitor rounding the sidewalk—our local congressman, Roscoe Bartlett.

A few moments later, he interrupted our meeting in the commander's office. I had met Congressman Bartlett on a couple of occasions, and he usually has a folksy, farm-boy manner. Not today. Fort Detrick fell within his district, and he had read our press release. He launched into a tirade, accusing us of creating a firestorm over nothing.

"If you took soil samples around Frederick County, you would probably find anthrax everywhere," he complained. "I probably have some on my boots."

The commander spent the next half hour calmly and painstakingly explaining the situation and our response.

To prove his point, before leaving, the congressman reached into his pocket and pulled out a clear glass jar, the size of a prescription bottle, filled with a dark brown substance. "I brought some dirt from my farm," he said as he set the bottle on the end of the conference table. "I want you to test this for anthrax."[3]

The commander reluctantly agreed to do so.

Shortly thereafter the commander concluded the meeting, saying he would order a formal "15–6" army investigation into possible wrongdoing in how the building contamination occurred and why a single researcher took it upon himself to do sampling of his office. 15–6 investigations are never fun. Usually some poor sucker, a military officer or government civilian external to the situation, gets appointed as the investigating officer. A colonel from our sister institute, the Walter Reed Army Institute of Research, was directed to investigate. He called me and many others to provide sworn testimony for his report.

Unfortunately, the building contamination occurred near simultaneously with another event, which did little to reassure the public of our competence. About ten days earlier, an anthrax researcher and technician had come to our clinic because they worried about a possible exposure to anthrax.[4] We routinely evaluated anyone who had a mishap in the containment laboratories. Most were minor.

Not this one.

Scientists who work on anthrax occasionally grow organisms to test them in the lab. The scientists injected some bacteria into a liquid broth and then incubated the solution overnight in two-liter flasks that swirled to mix in air for optimal growth. According to the standard procedure, one of the scientists screwed the lids on tight and then loosened them back a quarter turn to allow air exchange. He then taped a paper towel and gauze over the lid. The next morning he opened the flasks inside a biosafety hood and removed the paper towels and gauze. When he discarded the gauze and towels in the garbage next to him just outside the hood, the scientist noted some dried liquid on the paper towels, the neck of the flasks, and the screw tops. Somehow, some of the broth had spilled out over the top of the flasks, like a bubbling volcano, and dripped down the necks.

He was worried—and for good reason.

An air curtain flows continuously down across the front of a biosafety hood to protect the lab worker from the organisms inside. However, when the researcher pulled the paper towels and gauze out of the hood through the air curtain, it could have provided the energy source to spray anthrax spores into the air—like putting talcum powder in front of a fan. Neither of the scientists wore respiratory protection at the time, since they would have been vaccinated.

Each containment lab suite is divided into a series of labs off a central corridor, which function like individual vacuum "containers." Within minutes any contamination in the air would be sucked up and filtered safely out of the air. No one in the neighboring rooms had any risk, but the two scientists with the anthrax flasks stood at ground zero. They could have inhaled any spores floating in the air and developed the "queen mother" of the anthrax infections: inhalational anthrax.

When Ellen Boudreau, my clinic chief physician, evaluated the two scientists, she was worried. Large exposures to a pathogen can overwhelm the protection from any vaccine. She started them on the antibiotic ciprofloxacin as a preventive measure, just in case. She also swabbed their noses to test for anthrax spores. Whenever treatment was prescribed for a possible lab exposure, we sent a summary to the army's safety headquarters. This occasionally led to increased scrutiny from the media or the army chain of command, including at times, orders for the institute to conduct a "safety stand down."

In this situation the proximity in time with the hallway contamination hurt us. Media reports sounded as if the two lab workers had been exposed to anthrax *because* of the building contamination. That was wrong. They were two separate incidents.[5] The anthrax in the lab exposure carried a resistance marker to distinguish it from other strains.

These two events occurred while we had been running 24/7 operations in our Special Pathogens Lab for months to assess thousands of FBI samples, letters sent to Senators Daschle and Leahy, and samples from the contaminated Hart Senate office building. Sadly, at its finest hour, as USAMRIID supported the national anthrax response effort, the institute commander had to stand in front of the workforce in the Fort Detrick gym to reassure everyone that "USAMRIID is safe." Somehow it didn't seem right, but as that same commander once told me after another disaster, "It is what it is." We dealt with it and marched forward the best we could.

The local town of Frederick, Maryland, has a love-hate relationship with Fort Detrick. Fort Detrick is the largest local employer, but the local paper frequently criticizes the base for events like this one. Although we tried to be proactive to maintain good relations, the institute commander still had to do a mea culpa to the Frederick mayor during a press conference.

When the FBI later named a former USAMRIID researcher, Dr. Steven Hatfill, as a "person of interest" in their investigation of the anthrax letter attacks, suspicion that the perpetrator of the attacks might have come from within USAMRIID cast another shadow over the institute's efforts, making the institute "radioactive." After the anthrax letter attacks quieted down, we were chagrined that President Bush flew down to Atlanta to congratulate the CDC for its efforts. We never saw him, even though we were an hour up the road from the White House. After several months the army surgeon general paid us a visit, but it was too little too late. The entire institute staff assembled in the Fort Detrick gym for over an hour waiting for his entourage to arrive. He spent most of his time at the Fort Detrick headquarters and then did a short appearance for a few words before departing quickly. The deputy commander from our higher headquarters handed out the congratulatory certificates, instead, to all the "unsung heroes" who had assisted with the diagnostics response effort.

In 2008 the press covered the army's official 15–6 investigation when the 361-page report was released through a Freedom of Information Act request.[6] Some of the conclusions focused on adherence and documentation of safety procedures supervision. Recommendations included the need for better reporting procedures for biological mishaps, improved written precautions for lab procedures, regular retraining, and lab inspections.

One key conclusion the report could not make was the source of the contamination. It suggested the possibility of inadequate decontamination of containers brought out of lab suite B-3 or from the opening of evidentiary material from the FBI there, such as the letters and other items contaminated with powdered anthrax. Jeff Adamovicz, deputy chief of Bacteriology, who had come up with a technique months earlier to quantitate the spore concentrations in the anthrax letters, had expressed concern about the risk of contamination in the hallway months earlier. Those concerns may now have been realized, but ironically he felt the brunt of the blame. The hallway contamination led to finger-pointing between the different divisions in USAMRIID that worked on anthrax and supported the investigation––who was at fault?

This event was only the beginning of more challenges to come. Dr. Bruce Ivins, the anthrax expert who did the unauthorized testing in his office, justified doing so because one of his contract technicians worried about potential exposure to powdered spores from the letters. Ivins noted that his desk had been covered in dirt and dust by others temporarily using his office. He had done some earlier testing of his desk back in December 2001 and found growth consistent with anthrax. At the time Dr. Ivins decontaminated areas around his desk but did nothing further to confirm the results, nor did he notify his superiors. His boss, the Bacteriology Division chief, was reprimanded because of it, but colleague and bacteriologist Hank

Heine argued that "Bruce was completely within his rights to do that, because it was a safety situation. If he suspected there was contamination, he was right to get down there with some swabs and figure out what was going on."

Jeff Adamovicz said that years later, when the FBI would focus its attention on Bruce Ivins as the possible anthrax letter perpetrator, it would use his taking of swab samples in his office against him, asserting, "He's covering up the evidence of malfeasance." On the contrary, Jeff believes "it could've also been that in fact what he [Bruce] claimed was actually correct . . . but that never really got resolved."

In 2002 the FBI investigation was still in its infancy, but it would dog the institute for years to come.

The nose sample from one of the two scientists exposed in the lab came back positive, confirming our worst fears that anthrax spores in the fluid that had trickled out of the neck of the two-liter flasks had gone airborne. Ellen Boudreau had made the right judgment call to start the scientists on antibiotics.

To our relief, though, everything in the laundry facility came up clean. I had a follow-up phone call with the manager there, who was satisfied with our response.

We tested the soil sample from the congressman's farm. The result: negative for anthrax.

The hallway contamination experience pulled me into the leadership cadre of the institute more effectively than any prior experience, because our quick response seeing the workforce in the Medical Division was critical to quelling what could have been a much bigger disaster. Although it came the hard way, I could also add risk communication to my new set of skills.

At this point for me, anthrax went into the rearview mirror. I had to shift my focus back to vaccinating the forces because the pendulum had swung toward war with Iraq, focused on Saddam Hussein's biological weapons caches. Smallpox was at the heart of those concerns.

Bow to King Smallpox

In the 1700s anyone alive knew that he or she would someday face King Smallpox. Once infected, a person had a 30 percent chance of dying, but even survivors might end up blind, deformed, or with permanent scars all over their bodies.

The normal attack route came through infected droplets landing on the membranes in the nose or mouth, but different civilizations learned that exposing people to the virus in other ways could prevent the disease. Some blew scabs from smallpox victims up their noses or took a scab or pus from an oozing smallpox lesion and scraped it onto someone's arm. This process, called variolation, prevented illness in most, but because it used the same deadly virus, it risked giving the recipient smallpox disease instead. Between 1 and 3 percent of those who had received variolation died.

Edward Jenner, an English country doctor, observed that milkmaids had beautiful skin—at a time when smallpox left most people with pockmarked faces. He wondered whether the mild pustules milkmaids got on their hands from cowpox, a similar infection in cows, protected them against smallpox. He decided to test this theory on eight-year-old James Phipps, who was due to receive variolation. Jenner substituted some cowpox pus from a milkmaid instead of smallpox and scraped it onto James's arm. Over the next several days, James developed a pustule from the cowpox. A couple of weeks later, Jenner tried it again but replaced cowpox with the actual smallpox virus (variolation) instead. This time James had no pustular response—the cowpox infection had made him immune to smallpox. Jenner then performed the same test on twenty-three other people. Success. He wrote up his findings. Despite initial skepticism from his medical colleagues, Jenner's work gave birth to the first "vaccine" (from the Latin, *vacca*, for cow). Cowpox vaccination was adopted as a safer alternative to variolation. Jenner realized the significance of his 1796 finding, writing in a subsequent report, "It now becomes too manifest to admit of controversy, that the annihilation of the Small Pox, the most dreadful scourge of the human species, must be the final result of this practice."[1]

Vaccination was the core of smallpox control and ultimately led to WHO's global effort centuries later to wipe smallpox off the face of the earth. In 1980, when the World Health Assembly officially announced the eradication of smallpox, it asked all countries to turn their stocks of smallpox virus into repositories at the CDC or in the Soviet Union. After that, countries gradually stopped vaccinating against smallpox.

The unfortunate, unanticipated outcome of this public-health triumph was that as populations lost their immunity over time, smallpox's attractiveness as a bioweapon increased. We at USAMRIID had been ringing alarm bells about smallpox for years, and our scientists initiated projects to develop new treatments and vaccines. Others began to take notice of the threat, which took many forms.

Had all countries really surrendered their smallpox stocks back in 1980, especially those that sponsor terrorism? What if someone unearthed smallpox from victims frozen in the permafrost or genetically engineered a new smallpox virus from a related virus or from scratch?

Understanding what happened in a *vaccinated* population in the former Yugoslavia provided a chilling example of smallpox's potential. In 1972 a Yugoslavian man traveled on a pilgrimage to Mecca. On his way home, he passed through Iraq, where smallpox still occurred. After arriving home he may have felt ill but still invited friends over to tell them about his trip. Within two weeks eleven people developed smallpox—all unrecognized. Two weeks later over 150 more cases of smallpox exploded. The Yugoslavian government took extreme measures to shut down the epidemic by closing the borders, locking up the victims in a hotel in Sarajevo, and vaccinating the entire population of the country.

After the first Gulf War (1990–91), Iraq admitted that it had done research on camel pox virus—a close cousin to smallpox that causes disease in camels. Did Iraq intend to genetically engineer camel pox to make it act like smallpox? If the United States launched an invasion into Iraq, would Saddam Hussein unleash smallpox on U.S. forces or on the U.S. homeland?

We had no idea, but immediately after the anthrax letters of 2001, mindful of smallpox's long reach and deadly capabilities, countries around the world scrambled for smallpox vaccine. By then the United States only had 15.3 million doses available for a population of over 280 million.

As the U.S. war machine started preparing for war with Iraq, the White House took notice of the specter of a weaponized smallpox attack. Vice President Dick Cheney pushed hard for action, and the CDC began to offer smallpox vaccine to civilian health-care providers, despite pushback from medical authorities. DoD preparations also kicked into gear.

Colonel Charles Hoke, an army infectious disease doctor with light brown hair and a boyish grin, ran the program that funded infectious disease research in military laboratories. His long, distinguished career included a tour with the CDC's Epidemic Intelligence Service and running research studies in Thailand on dengue fever, Japanese encephalitis, and influenza. On a Thursday afternoon in July 2002, he received the dreaded phone call from his boss, the chief of Staff to the commanding general at Fort Detrick's headquarters, that every military officer knows can come at any time.

"Colonel Hoke. You have been selected to be the army's representative on the Select Agents Response Task Force (SARTF), and you will report for duty at the Office of the Surgeon General on Tuesday next week." Colonel Hoke argued that he was essential in his current job and couldn't leave, adding, "I will need to hear this from the general." The general got on the phone. "Yes, Colonel Hoke, those are my instructions." Colonel Hoke asked, "Do you have any special guidance?" "Yes," the general responded, "do the best job you can."

Colonel Hoke hung up and immediately placed a call to an old friend at the surgeon general's office. "Is there any way I can get out of this assignment?" Colonel Hoke asked. "No problem, Charles," his friend told him. "All you need to do is convince the commanding general of MRMC [Medical Research and Materiel Command], the head of the Army Medical Department, and the surgeon general that someone else is better qualified, and you're free."

Colonel Hoke relented.

On Monday he cleared out his office at Fort Detrick. On Tuesday he reported to the army surgeon general's office to support Colonel John Grabenstein at the SARTF, whose primary mission was developing a plan to protect U.S. forces from smallpox. A key element: immunize U.S. forces in advance of an anticipated invasion of Iraq. John Grabenstein, a pharmacist with a broad forehead, steel-blue eyes, and a presidential look reminiscent of John Quincy Adams, was the right man to lead the SARTF. He brought a laser focus to the SARTF after spending the prior two years running the army's anthrax vaccination program.

John said, "We're just moving papers as fast as we can do it and trying to get everything put together," and one day Dr. Hoke and another medical colleague showed up, "briefcases in hand" at the cubicle farm supporting the army surgeon general and said, "We're here for the SARTF." John asked, "What's that?" Apparently, no one had bothered to inform him that he was in charge of the SARTF. Nevertheless, Dr. Hoke had a piece of paper authorizing him to be there, so John put him to work.

Once on board Dr. Hoke immediately understood the stakes. Not only was there a threat to the Unites States' completely susceptible military population, but the safety of the homeland was also at stake. Soldiers infected on the battlefield risked bringing the virus home and lighting the flame that could spread a wildfire across the United States and to the world beyond.

But vaccinating the U.S. military forces had just gotten harder. In the late fall of 2001, Wyeth Pharmaceuticals lost its license for the vaccine, even though it had considerable quantities of vaccine in storage. The smallpox vaccine has three components: the dried vaccine in a vial; a second, smaller vial containing liquid (the diluent), which mixes with the vaccine to liquefy it for vaccination; and a two-and-one-half-inch-long specialized needle (the bifurcated needle) that looks like a miniature, two-pronged pitchfork. Unless all the components are functional, the vaccine can't be used. In 2001 the diluent became the Achilles heel when it failed testing.

Overnight, no one inside or outside of the military could use the vaccine, even though the vaccine itself still worked. The Office of the Vice President pushed strongly to get a new vaccine into the national stockpile, but until a new diluent and bifurcated needles could be remanufactured, the vaccine became "investigational," subject to all the FDA's rigorous requirements for conducting a research study.

Just like Jenner had done in the 1700s, the smallpox vaccine is still administered differently than other vaccines. Instead of being injected deep into the muscle with a long needle, the bifurcated needle is dipped into the vaccine solution, and it captures the exact amount of liquid in between its two tiny prongs to give a single vaccine dose. The vaccinator then wipes the liquid on the upper arm and pierces the skin multiple times with the needle at the same location to carry the vaccine into the skin with each penetration. Over the next week or so, the live virus in the vaccine replicates in the skin, and the patient develops a pus-filled blister at the site, like eight-year old James Phipps developed in the 1700s. This blister is a good sign: it indicates that the patient has a "take" and is therefore becoming immune. A scar eventually develops, leaving a permanent record of successful vaccination.

My division at USAMRIID joined the smallpox vaccine preparation effort because giving the vaccine was a unique skill set that few people still had back in 2001. We were the only place in the DoD and one of the few in the country with any recent experience giving smallpox vaccine, because we gave it to our lab workers conducting research on monkeypox and smallpox.[2]

While the SARTF continued with its preparations, the Armed Forces Epidemiology Board (AFEB), a highly respected scientific advisory panel for the DoD made up of civilian experts, weighed in and endorsed "the development of policies and contingency plans for use of smallpox vaccine for military personnel." The AFEB also noted that "any use of investigational smallpox vaccine should be done on a voluntary basis."

That sounded great—on the surface. Giving a licensed vaccine to the forces is easy. Soldiers in basic training are like pincushions and get loads of them. Line them up, roll up their sleeves, and inject them "double barreled" in both arms in a human assembly line. "Investigational products" are different. They come wrapped in red tape with a whole different set of rules—and paperwork. It's not like issuing flak jackets. We cannot force soldiers to take them—not even in the military. Every soldier must read and sign a two-dozen-page consent form—and that's after you have sat them down and presented the vaccine's risks and benefits. It's hard to imagine adhering to this legal procedure while dodging enemy bullets. Soldiers had the right to refuse—even when facing an imminent threat. Such a complex process is no way to protect an army.

Dr. Hoke blasted me and a couple of USAMRIID colleagues an urgent note on July 16 about the march toward vaccinating the forces with an investigational product, stressing, "I'm trying to keep on the table that there is a vast difference between what can be done now [with an unlicensed vaccine] and [later] once there is a licensed vaccine. As hard as I try, there is the most incredible pressure to come up with a plan." The SARTF was moving forward with the assumption that the vaccine would be relicensed in time for the war, but the team had to develop a contingency plan just in case there was a glitch. "Shit happens" is a way of life in the military, and things going wrong has to be part of the daily calculations.

Among ourselves and the SARTF, we discussed the possible need to request a presidential waiver of informed consent; otherwise, we couldn't guarantee protection of the forces. Those of us at USAMRIID just didn't believe that the decision makers at the highest level understood the challenge of what they were asking for—vaccinating the forces with an investigational vaccine—but we also knew that having the president waive informed consent was unlikely because it would be a political death trap.

The military generally tries to align its policies for protecting the health and autonomy of soldiers with civilian public health organizations like the CDC and the FDA, but occasionally, war operations present unique challenges without simple solutions. The military and the FDA had been burned before, during the first Gulf War, when soldiers were injected with vaccines without knowing what they were receiving. The specter of Gulf War Syndrome loomed

Bow to King Smallpox

over the effort, because vaccines had been considered a potential cause of that illness until they were later discounted. John Grabenstein at the SARTF knew that if the DoD had to vaccinate soldiers with an IND vaccine, it had to do it right. He said, "There was never any discussion of 'we'll give them a one-page summary, or we'll hoodwink them, we'll try and pull the wool over their eyes'; there was always respect for informed consent." The main issue was how that could be achieved, but there was no good way to handle all the required FDA paperwork and tracking who got vaccinated. John recalls thinking, "Imagine if it's a ten- or twenty-page consent form and it's a half a million people, so how many pages is that and what are we going to do with all that paper?" For five hundred thousand soldiers, a twenty-pager translates to ten million pages, twenty thousand reams, and fifty tons of twenty-pound bond paper! There were no portable electronic solutions then.

The chief of the Allergy-Immunology Department at Walter Reed's National Vaccine Healthcare Center emailed that she had "grave concerns about the implementation issues . . . making anthrax [vaccine] look like kindergarten" compared with smallpox vaccine. "The risk of failure, if not done in a way that facilitates compliance and success, is high. . . . We have the potential to lose a lot of trust in vaccine programs in general if we do not do this right."

My colleagues at our sister lab, the Walter Reed Army Institute of Research (WRAIR), put it even more bluntly: "The assumption that this entire process can be accomplished under the rubric of a clinical research protocol is flawed. . . . The IND regulations are not intended for mass public health interventions of the type envisioned by this plan."

The DoD drove on anyway, but Colonel Hoke did his best to sound a note of caution to the planners.

On August 24, 2002, the army surgeon general signed a memo directing our command to develop a protocol to dilute the existing smallpox vaccine fivefold, which could expand the limited national stockpile. We took on this task, along with our other contingency vaccine protocols. USAMRIID's higher-level command was further directed to prepare a plan to vaccinate one thousand volunteers, with an expansion to thirty-thousand, if needed.[3]

But this small number would not solve the problem for the DoD. Vaccinating one thousand volunteers is one thing. Trying to vaccinate half a million forces with an investigational product would spell disaster, but waiting for a licensed vaccine would take time. We didn't have time to wait, which risked delaying the launch date for war in the Iraqi desert into the middle of the summer. That would be a problem.

With leadership from the White House and the Office of the Vice President, in consultation with experts such as Dr. D. A. Henderson, who led the global smallpox eradication effort, and retired army major general Philip Russell, a respected scientist and vaccine developer, who met frequently with the vice president, the pieces led by the SARTF began to fall into place. Colonel Hoke started to get some traction with the challenges and risks of using an investigational vaccine. The DoD joined forces with the FDA and Wyeth. As Phil Russell said, "We pushed really hard [on Wyeth], and they went all out to bring those lots out of deep storage and get them approved for use." Wyeth assigned a former army physician-scientist to lead the effort to methodically conduct studies and assemble the documents and information needed to get the vaccine relicensed. The Wyeth team worked around the clock, and the FDA reviewed the documents from them in real time. But John Grabenstein is quick to point out that "nobody ever brought undue influence on the FDA." Phil Russell said, "At that point in time, interagency differences were set aside. Everybody was on the same page and wanted to get the jobs done."

On September 12 a new directive came from the Pentagon to form smallpox epidemiologic response teams and treatment teams. I worked with the USAMRIID commander to assign our different docs, nurses, and technicians to the respective teams.

The SARTF's preparedness effort culminated in organizing a "DoD Smallpox Preparedness Conference" for the team members from October 29 to November 1, 2002, in a hotel near the Pentagon. Masterfully orchestrated to fly under the media radar, hundreds of DoD medical personnel from around the country converged for training on smallpox recognition, learning how to vaccinate, managing vaccine reactions, and getting vaccinated themselves. Our USAMRIID nurses gave hands-on training, while vaccinating the care providers. I lectured to a hotel ballroom full of military docs and nurses from the army, navy, and air force on how to vaccinate using an investigational protocol. Even as I lectured, I couldn't help thinking that this was a fool's errand. I just wasn't convinced that we could pull off vaccinating an invasion force with an investigational vaccine. There had to be a better way.

John Grabenstein recalls, "We were living, eating, and breathing biodefense stuff, contingency planning, but there remained a concern that if they couldn't get a presidential waiver and they had to give the vaccine under IND, how could they do it? Well, you then need some specialists, dedicated people who can do the training, . . . explain the risks and benefits," and accomplish all the other tasks of giving an IND vaccine. At a meeting one afternoon, John said that a Specialized Medical Augmentation and Response Team (SMART) for biodefense was needed to do this.

As the winter of 2002 arrived, the DoD figured out its "better way." John's idea of a SMART team took hold. The army was scouting for a field-ready "dream team" of experienced medical officers who understood infectious diseases, bioweapons, investigational vaccines, and how to give them. War preparations continued, but the work on a smallpox vaccine was only the beginning.

In my mind I heard the unmistakable, ominous "WHOP-WHOP-WHOP" sound of Blackhawk helicopters just over the horizon. They were coming for me.

12

On the Front Lines

··

Gas! GAS! Quick, boys!—An ecstasy of fumbling
Fitting the clumsy helmets just in time,
But someone still was yelling out and stumbling
And flound'ring like a man in fire or lime.—
Dim through the misty panes and thick green light,
As under a green sea, I saw him drowning.
In all my dreams before my helpless sight,
He plunges at me, guttering, choking, drowning.

—from "Dulce et decorum est," by Wilfred Owen, a World War I poem depicting
the horror of gas trench warfare

CAMP DOHA, KUWAIT CITY. 1:30 A.M. MARCH 28, 2003

Nine days after the bombs of "shock and awe" rained down on Iraq, a shock wave shuddered through the desert warehouse where I was dead asleep on a cot. The explosion jolted me wide-awake along with hundreds of other sleeping soldiers. A clatter rippled overhead as roof tiles collided in succession like dominoes, and the concrete floor trembled.

"What . . . the FUCK . . . was THAT!?" a deep voice yelled.

"EVERYBODY OUT! NOW!"

Bodies everywhere erupted from sleep in the "The Cave," our living quarters in an open-bay warehouse the size of an airplane hangar.

Shit, I thought. *A Scud missile?! We're under attack.*

I fumbled in the dark under my cot for my chemical protective suit and gas mask, which I kept within reach at all times, yanking them on as I stumbled out of the dusty warehouse and into the cool, clear night. Outside was chaos and sensory overload: the buzzing generators and bright floodlights made it hard to think through my sleepy fog.

A river of masked soldiers, like extras in a sci-fi movie, streamed into concrete bunkers just a few steps from The Cave. I entered one the size of an airport shuttle, and we kept packing in bodies—twenty or thirty until we overflowed the space. Then I waited, in anticipation, hearing others around me sucking wind in their masks. Our base on the outskirts of Kuwait City was the nerve center for the United States during Operation Iraqi Freedom. We were a prime target. Were other bombs incoming?

After years building my foundational skills in the hospital and running the lab response side of germ-warfare defense, I sat poised on the front lines, crammed shoulder to shoulder, with other soldiers wearing M90 gas masks that would give some people nightmares, but they were our last line of defense against nerve agents and infectious viruses and bacteria spread by aerosol. I was here to protect these soldiers from the invisible living agents that could be unleashed by those bombs, which could take days to identify. For some that would be too late. This felt like the midterm exam of my career.

There was nothing I could do in the bunker but wait, think, and breathe, which was a struggle in and of itself. Sucking air into an M90 gas mask takes breathing power, and when you're already out of breath it feels suffocating. The harder I breathed, the more claustrophobic I felt, and the deeper the panic set in. Shaking from adrenaline, I braced for the next bomb, fearing it would be filled with nerve agent—or worse.

We had reason to be afraid. Despite signing the 1972 Biological Weapons Convention, a worldwide treaty to end the production and storage of weapons-grade germs, Iraq had admitted in 1995 to developing and stockpiling tons of chemical and biological weapons for tactical use during the first Gulf War.[1] Anthrax. Botulinum toxin. Aflatoxin, a poisonous toxin produced by mold. Iraq had also used chemical weapons against Iran during their war in the 1980s. There was no reason to assume that Iraq did not have them still, thirteen years after the 1990 Gulf War, "Operation Desert Shield/Storm."

As part of its defense strategy and the culmination of our contingency protocol and smallpox vaccine efforts, the U.S. military had deployed me on an A-team of nine chemical and biological warfare experts. Working and traveling as our own independent unit, we had a mission to vaccinate troops against the biological agent presumed most likely to be used against us by Saddam Hussein: botulinum toxin. We transported hundreds of vials of treatments and antitoxins, a delicate arsenal of countermeasures that we had to keep cold at all times, lest they expire in the desert heat. We had a short timeline to disseminate these countermeasures to several military field hospitals and medical centers in Kuwait, and train medical personnel on how to administer them before the launch of the invasion force. The number of potential victims was staggering: around 130,000 American troops were dispatched during the initial invasion of Iraq. Our supplies would be enough to treat only a tiny fraction of them.

There are many ways to die at war, but I can imagine few ways more horrific than death by a nerve agent or botulinum toxin (bot). If you had to choose between the two, it's a toss-up.

Nerve agents, as the name implies, attack our body's nerve network, which buzzes in constant communication. Each nerve strand transmits messages throughout the body—"Breathe." "Smile." "Duck!"—through chemical "ferries" (signals) passed across channels from one neuron to the next. A single drop of vx liquid will penetrate the skin rapidly and trigger a flood of chemical transmitters into those tiny channels, causing hyperstimulation. Like the frantic writhing of a wasp after you spray it with Raid, the nerves go haywire, bombarded with unceasing messages that cause you to lose control of your body in all the worst ways: drooling, vomiting, losing bowel control, and ultimately seizing—before you stop breathing.[2] The only bit of good news is that by the time you seize, at least you don't know what's happening.

Botulinum toxin causes the opposite effect, paralysis, by blocking the chemical signal "ferries" leaving the nerve port. It starts with your head and moves down. First comes blurry or double vision. Next comes trouble swallowing. You might notice your voice sounds funny, or maybe you start choking. Your eyelids sag, your head droops, and your face looks dazed and zombielike as your facial muscles become slack. The worst part is that your mind stays alert, but you cannot speak. You are fully conscious as you suffocate.

Taking a bullet seems more appealing.

My team's mission to protect our troops from this kind of horrific demise had begun months earlier back at Fort Detrick, Maryland. Dubbed the SMART-IND (Special Medical Augmentation and Response Team for Investigational New Drugs) team, our group was created by the army surgeon general in late 2002—a "dream team" of military infectious disease doctors, research nurses, and support technicians. With a short lead time to war, we launched something akin to the Manhattan Project of biodefense on the fringes of Fort Detrick in a double-wide trailer with lopsided floors and stained carpets, and without fanfare but with direct access to the senior military leadership. Our mission: to develop field-ready protocols—basically rules of engagement—governing the use of unlicensed vaccines and antidotes for biological warfare.[3]

Shortly after our work began, we received a gift. In record time all the work by Colonels John Grabenstein and Charles Hoke at the SARTF, Wyeth Pharmaceuticals, and the FDA paid off. By December 16, 2002, two lots of smallpox vaccine were approved for use with a new diluent. Now we had a licensed vaccine against smallpox. In short order the military did what it does best, vaccinating over five hundred thousand military personnel against smallpox, which knocked King Smallpox off his throne as the top threat. Similarly, the anthrax vaccination of the forces hobbled Queen Anthrax.

This left "bot" (botulinum toxin) as our top threat. We had a vaccine and treatments to defend against bot, but none were licensed by the FDA. We had to cut through the FDA red tape and teach others how to use these "investigational products," but it's not so simple adhering to the FDA's requirements with incoming Scud missiles raining from the sky.

It might seem tempting to "lose" the paperwork somewhere in the desert. But ignoring the FDA's rules was not a viable option and could cost us our careers. Gulf War Syndrome had dogged the military after the first Gulf war. Part of our mission was to prevent Gulf War Syndrome, Part 2.

Al Magill, our most senior doc on the team, had a Teddy bear personality, a playful smile, and a gift for telling senior leaders the truth in simple, unvarnished terms. He briefed our commanding general at Fort Detrick one afternoon, wagging his right index finger to emphasize the point: "Sir, whoever signs the 1572 [a form, signed by the lead investigator, that binds an investigator to protect human subjects] no longer works for you. They work for the FDA." Meeting the FDA's requirements was an impossible task in a war environment and the crux of our challenge. The general understood. He assured us that the in-country leader would get us what we needed to do this right.

Not only were we hog-tied with legal regulations, but our vaccines had been sitting in storage for decades. *Decades!* Like most medicines these products have a limited shelf life, and their effectiveness declines over time. Some of the products had problems we could work around. One botulinum antitoxin treatment had developed protein clumps that interfered with its usual intravenous delivery. We proposed injecting it into muscles as a preventive measure instead. Other instances were fraught with irony. The FDA did not want us to offer the botulism vaccine to soldiers because recent tests showed its protection in mice and guinea pigs had waned for some of the five serotypes in the vaccine. That made no sense to us trying to protect our soldiers and marines. Wasn't partial protection still better than none at all?

I raised this question at a meeting with the FDA. "How, in good conscience, can you deny these potentially lifesaving products for our forces?" I asked.

The FDA department chief snapped back, jabbing her finger at me. "You can't put that on us. We told you [the DoD] to make a new vaccine ten years ago."

She was right. It was embarrassing and idiotic. Thirteen years after Operation Desert Storm, we were still talking about the same outdated bot vaccine. A newer one was in the pipeline but years away from becoming licensed. The army channeled money only to certain products and priorities, many of which were never on the radar for development for civilians.

After a brief hiatus, the FDA eventually relented, and the bot vaccine was back on the table.

Ironically, some of our fellow military members gave our team pushback and made us feel like stepchildren. Shortly before we shipped off to the desert, we were told that the lead medical general in-theater wanted to split us up and send some of us to work in a clinic in Qatar. We needed adequate numbers of team members. Splitting us up would guarantee mission failure. But even generals have bosses. The winds shifted again, and we learned that Vice President Cheney was tracking our mission. We were told our team would stay intact.

We nonetheless often found ourselves at odds with other high-ranking army officials. Before the invasion we met with the soldiers planning army operations (ops) deep in the bowels of the Pentagon. As my team members pitched our biodefense plan, the OPS guys didn't take us seriously. "You know, Colonel," one soldier said, "the time for good ideas has passed."

Even though biological and chemical weapons had by then become household concerns nationwide, it was challenging to convey the devastating power of microbes to officers accustomed to more concrete threats: bullets, tanks, and bombs. At times it was almost comical. Take, for instance, the meeting when another paper-pushing colonel in the Pentagon shut down my teammates, three senior infectious disease colonels, as they briefed him on the Iraqi bioweapons threat and our team's contingency plans for biowarfare.

"Stop right there," the colonel said, holding up his hands. My colleagues paused, confused. "Someone get me a tissue," the colonel said dryly, clearly mocking our concerns about a bioweapon attack. "I think I'm going to cry."

Our team leaders successfully explained their concerns, though, to Dr. Winkenwerder, the most senior physician in the DoD. Al Magill staged a battle scenario moving office supplies like chess pieces across a conference table representing an imaginary map of the Middle East.

"The problem, sir, is that the bad guys who want to do us harm are over here," Al said, placing a pen on imaginary Iraq. He slid a second object just south of the pen, indicating Kuwait. "Here are our vulnerable forces." He slid a third object to the other end of the world, over the United States. "The antidotes and the people who know how to give them [us] are over here," he said. "Ten thousand miles away."

Dr. Winkenwerder understood.

The next day, we learned we were going to war. Of the nineteen original members of the SMART-IND team, nine would deploy. We did not know who would draw the short straws or when they would be told. Not knowing was the hardest part.

The uncertainty had gnawed at me for the preceding two months of limbo as the team went on and off alert for possible deployment. I tried not to let on how I really felt and just dealt with it. At least we would have something definitive, I hoped, in the near future.

I distracted myself with standard prewar preparations: doctors' appointments for prescriptions, packing and repacking my duffle bags, and updating my will. I needed a smallpox vaccine, but I worried about exposing my wife and sons, who have eczema, which could lead to severe or even deadly reactions if they had contact with the potentially contagious virus. So instead of spending what could be my last few days at home, I checked into a motel with stained carpets and a broken heater to wait out the period when the vaccine had the highest risk of spread. On my tenth night in the motel, I was half asleep when the phone rang.

"Mark," the voice said, "you are one of the ones deploying. We're sorry." "Okay," I mumbled, in a partial dream state but feeling the weight of the news. "I understand."

Iraqi Freedom was not my first deployment. Years earlier I had deployed for nine months to Bosnia as the chief of Preventive Medicine for the U.S. forces. Although I put in a lot of miles in a Humvee on dangerous roadways and occasional hostile surroundings assessing our bases around the country, it was a peacekeeping mission.

The specter of war felt different.

I felt a strange cocktail of guilt and excitement. This was the adventure of a lifetime, an opportunity I looked forward to and had prepared for my whole career, but I hated leaving my family. My wife, Cindy, was six-months pregnant. Ten-year-old Luke was a baseball player, beginning to play the piano and the violin. Four-year-old Sean was still in preschool, a cuddly armful with a killer smile. I still held him every night as he fell asleep.

Because our team was a fringe element and not deploying with a massive military unit, Cindy lacked the support other military wives would have during a typical deployment. She was particularly upset that she couldn't ask our church to pray for me, because we were told not to broadcast our activities—the old "loose lips sink ships" adage.

I feared I would miss the birth of my third son. I had bonded with his little form on ultrasound, and we had picked out a name, Daniel. I worried I might never meet him. At the same time, I had mixed feelings about the challenges of becoming a father for the third time. After ten years and two boys, I enjoyed the increasing freedom and felt some reluctance about changing diapers again but also guilty for feeling that way. In some ways deploying allowed me to escape dealing with my own reality back home.

The night before I was due to ship out, after we tucked the boys in, Cindy and I were lying in bed, talking quietly.

"I'm afraid I might not come back this time," I said, choking on the words.

Cindy did not cry, but just held me. Strong as she is, physically and emotionally, she would later confess how hard it was to ignore a belief she had that whenever there is a new birth in the family, someone dies.

Before I left home, I sat down at my desk and typed up a note for Cindy on the computer with financial instructions and a spreadsheet of all our accounts and passwords. I sealed it in an envelope, placed it in our home safe, and told Cindy where to find it. On the envelope I wrote, "Open if I don't return."

We shipped out to the Kuwaiti desert in late February. The deploying biodefense team included some of the military's finest infectious disease officers and researchers. Donald "Gray" Heppner led malaria vaccine research. Al Magill ran malaria drug research. Chris Ockenhouse was a gifted malaria lab scientist. Robert Kuschner, our team leader, was an expert on a range of diseases of military importance.[4] Even though I was a department chief at the largest biodefense lab in the world, they all outranked me and were legendary in the military infectious disease community. As the junior physician on the team and with less research experience, I felt a little out of my league.

At Camp Doha, near Kuwait City, we set up our team headquarters in a one-room office, around 220 square feet, where all nine team members worked closely—literally and figuratively. Our office sat in prime real estate in the Command Center—the "Forbidden City," as Gray Heppner, our philosophical team member who often quoted literature, called it. An island in a sea of warehouses with special access restrictions and isolated from the rest of the base by a closely monitored boundary of razor wire, the Command Center ran all in-theater military operations.

We had shipped ourselves a whole bunch of supplies: an industrial-strength printer for the paperwork and about twenty green foot-lockers set up as "go boxes." These trunks contained a few hundred freezer bags prepackaged with everything needed to administer one treatment course of botulinum antitoxin: needles, syringes, intravenous tubing, IV catheters, and alcohol and gauze pads. If we got an emergency midnight call, we could grab the footlockers, hop on a chopper, and be ready to treat upon arrival within minutes.

The actual botulinum antidotes and vaccines arrived separately in specialized cold containers called Vaxicools. The size of a large suitcase, these portable battery-powered refrigerators can hold up to four hundred vials of antitoxin.

Many things that we take for granted back home are nearly impossible to find in a war zone. Just picking up the vaccines and antitoxins at the airport required a 3:00 a.m. convoy, a search around the airport maze, and a lengthy negotiation with customs.

We also needed a secure location with a power source to keep the products cold. It seems so basic, but electrical outlets don't sprout from the desert sand. We approached the on-base medical clinic, but we received a lukewarm reception. They had enough challenges with war casualty planning and caring for the routine sniffles, bumps, and bruises and wanted nothing to do with our products. Instead, we made nice with one of the third-country nationals who ran the medical warehouse to borrow some of their outlets for our freezer and the Vaxicools. The entire in-country supply of botulism counter-measures for our forces was kept alive by two electrical outlets in the warehouse. It was a perfect example of how the smallest detail could make or break an operation. A second fridge/freezer shipped to us disappeared in the "mail" on the way into the war zone, so we improvised and left most of the products in the Vaxicools, which were designed for transport, not for long-term storage.

The industrial-strength printer we brought was the single most important piece of equipment, spitting out thousands of pages of documents. One colleague estimated that if we had to treat the forces for botulism, the informed consent forms alone would weigh a ton or more.

Armed with medical products and the loathsome documents, in whatever limited time we had left, we were ready to launch our mission to train the U.S. docs in-country, thus multiplying the number of medical personnel who could assist us in responding to an attack with botulinum toxin.

We weren't convinced that our in-country leaders took the threat seriously. Others in the medical "cell" in-theater called us "prima donnas." We tried to get dedicated vehicles for our team, but we were rebuffed with empty promises. Ventilators that we thought were needed to save the most serious, paralyzed bot casualties never materialized.

When Bob Kuschner briefed the general about our mission—the same general who had wanted to split us up—Bob asked, "How many casualties are you expecting us to treat?" The general responded, "How many can you treat?" Bob provided a number. The general said, nonchalantly, "That's fine."

Though we worried about the worst-case scenario—a unit of hundreds of soldiers getting exposed to aerosolized bot—the simple things thwarted us daily.

One morning we planned to depart early in a three-vehicle convoy headed seventy kilometers north through the desert to Camp Udairi, Kuwait, which was the northernmost base near the Iraqi border. I did what I would do before any long drive—I checked the oil of my borrowed SUV. The dipstick was bone-dry. *Shit! Really?* I thought.

I refused to risk blowing my engine deep in the desert, but the base was an endless maze of warehouses, and it took some searching before I found the motor pool. The civilian employees there just shook their heads. "That's a contract vehicle," one said. "We can't give you oil. It's not our responsibility to provide oil for a contract suv." I thought, *What kind of bullshit policy is this?* but I said, "Are you kidding me?" "No."

The irony of being denied oil, by my own people, in a nation built on oil, was not lost on me. This was ridiculous. I pointed out the many barrels of oil stacked around the motor pool that could easily fill a tank battalion and told them they were impairing our mission. Begrudgingly, the employee gave me two quarts.

Exiting the base, we deliberately ran the red light where some contractors had been killed by sniper fire a few weeks earlier. It was surreal, passing the large pink and tan box-shaped houses that dotted the city landscape before civilization disappeared in an endless sea of sand.

A two-lane asphalt road served as the main artery going north. We wondered why none of the other vehicles driving in either direction used it. It didn't take too many spine-jarring potholes to figure out why, so we joined the others driving on the sand "highway."

We passed a roadside vehicle graveyard, sand welling in the pockets of the "victims'" twisted metal, when I realized we were driving on the so-called highway of death. At the end of the first Gulf War, the Iraqis retreated north along this very same road while the U.S. Air Force strafed and bombed the vehicles. In the resulting chaos, the gridlocked vehicles and occupants became sitting ducks. I gazed on the ghostlike ruins and could almost hear the echoes of screams and explosions.

As we cruised along at up to fifty miles per hour across the desert, I felt like Mad Max. We felt the hot, gritty heat of the day, despite the vehicle's air conditioning.

Camp Udairi, a vast tent city compound, emerged from the sand like a desert mirage. Our first order of business was a meeting with one of the operational units assigned to knock down the doors of potential biological weapon facilities in Iraq. The colonel in charge of this elite military unit had a very prominent bald forehead, giving him the nickname "Bullethead." He invited us to join him at his tactical operations center inside an armored personnel carrier.

We clambered upward through a two-inch-thick tank portal, which opened into a small meeting room. Surrounded by walls covered with operational maps and communications equipment, our team lead, Robert Kuschner, briefed Bullethead on Iraq's botulism threat and our antidotes and vaccines. We were all nervous, bracing for a chilly reception. Robert has a thin face, a shaved head, and a New York accent. He's usually a polished presenter, but this time his words came out a little shaky. A lot was at stake. We had to convince Bullethead to let us vaccinate his elite team.

Bullethead's posture, crossed arms, and frown suggested that he wasn't buying what we were selling. I had a sinking feeling as Robert flipped through his printed slide deck. Just a couple of slides into the brief, Bullethead stopped Robert, and I feared our five minutes were up. Instead, he leaned over to his executive officer and said: "Hey, can you get Bill in here?[5] He needs to hear this."

A few long minutes later, I was surprised to see a familiar face. Bill and I had worked together at Fort Detrick three years earlier. "My God, I didn't know you were here!" I said. "Great to see you!" he replied.

Bullethead warmed up considerably after that, and the tone of the meeting changed. By the time we left, we had exactly what we wanted: permission to offer our botulism vaccine and immune globulin to his soldiers on our next visit.

As we climbed down from the armored personnel carrier, the air had cooled, and the setting sun bathed the sand in a pink glow. I reflected on the amazing good fortune we had in the meeting. Maybe now we would be in business. The setting was peaceful in the moment, but I wondered what might lie beyond the horizon.

Our next stop was the Eighty-Sixth Combat Support Hospital (CSH) next door. In a few short days, when the bullets started strafing the sands, they would be the first mobile hospital to launch into Iraq. What we offered had direct relevance for their casualty preparations. The lead physician and twelve of his core medical staff listened attentively to my overview on how to recognize and treat botulism and smallpox. Government rules prohibited the physicians from giving the investigational bot treatment before they had been trained on the FDA regulations. So we left them cramming for an exam that would give them those credentials and then returned to our home base at Camp Doha. More intense training on the treatments would come on our next visit in a couple of days.

About five minutes from Camp Doha was a place called the Marble Palace, which was used for R&R. The sharp contrast with the desert gave it a Twilight Zone incongruity. An oasis of manicured grass and palm trees, the place had tinted windows under arches, marble floors, lounge chairs, tennis courts, putt-putt golf, and a swimming pool. It seemed like the furthest thing from war.

During a rare spell of down time, I sat by the pool and wrote a letter to Cindy:

> I am suspicious that it is only a matter of time before something happens. I just saw that Pres. Bush & Tony Blair arrived in the Azores to "discuss" options. I believe there is only one option they're discussing at this point, but you can read the papers as well as I & formulate your own conclusions. . . . By the time you get this, perhaps the war will already have started.
>
> I am not too concerned about something like a scud attack from where I am, although there is that possibility, I am more concerned about getting hit by a car on post or some other stupid accident, like being in a Blackhawk that goes down in a sandstorm. . . . I hope you're doing ok. I really miss feeling Daniel kick against your belly.

The next day, twenty minutes into the drive back to Camp Udairi, an alarm began beeping in the suv. I looked back to see the emergency lights flashing on the Vaxicool that held a large supply of antitoxin we were transporting. Its temperature was rising. We had plugged the Vaxicool into the suv's cigarette lighter, which must have shorted out. This was a serious problem. The priceless vials inside would be worthless if we couldn't maintain the proper temperature. Outside, the desert temperature was in the seventies and rising.

Chris Ockenhouse, an infectious disease doc with a long, thoughtful face and melancholy eyes, was in charge of the products. He rummaged around his backpack. "I think I have some batteries," he said.

We popped them in and held our breath. To our relief, the beeping stopped, and the temperatures recovered until we reached our destination. Another crisis averted.

It was March 17, 2003, one day before the "shock and awe" bombing began, but we did not know it then. We could sense the tension building, though. As we cruised northwest toward Camp Udairi, we passed endless convoys of desert-tan camouflaged tanks, armored personnel carriers, and Humvees packed with soldiers and duffle bags headed in the same direction: the Iraqi border. The U.S. military was mobilizing—and it was a sobering sight. I felt a mixture of pride and fear for what lay ahead.

When we arrived again at Camp Udairi, I plugged my laptop into a projector in a dusty hospital tent where I would give my presentation. A dozen or so doctors and nurses assembled in folding chairs to learn how to recognize smallpox and botulism and how to administer treatment. I projected my slides onto the tan canvas wall of the tent.

As I was in midsentence describing the Iraqi bioweapons program, my voice was drowned out by a siren. Like the haunting air raid sirens of World War II, it slowly crescendoed to a wailing pitch. This was the first time I had heard the sirens, and despite the desert heat, it gave me chills. "It permeates your bones," team member Gray Heppner said. We were under a Scud missile attack launched from across the border.

My audience and I instinctively tore open the Velcro flaps on our hips and pulled out our gas masks. Instead of ducking into the nearest bunker, as was protocol, I continued with my briefing, and my audience listened with rapt attention, even though I had to yell a little louder through the mask. I didn't feel particularly afraid of the Scuds, though I was probably naive, but the haunting siren scared me. Moments later the ground quaked as a battery of Patriot missiles launched to intercept the Scuds. It was a beautiful sound. Someone was protecting us. I didn't notice that one of my team members snapped a photo of me giving the brief through the gas mask. Behind me a photo of Saddam Hussein is projected against the canvas wall.

Next we prepared to vaccinate Bullethead's elite team, but not everyone opted in for the botulism vaccine or antitoxin. That was their choice. We couldn't make them volunteer, but the concept of not being able to require a potentially lifesaving measure still bothers me.

Set up in an empty ICU tent, we moved soldiers through the vaccination process like an assembly line: collecting medical histories, getting forms signed, and recording vital signs. Once all the administrative documents were done, we sent the soldiers behind a curtain, where our team nurse, Captain Jackie Carlin, was waiting, armed with syringes and long needles. No doubt some of the soldiers were surprised to find the petite brunette ready to give them the "Big Mac and fries." Jackie earned her pay that night, enduring flirting from the younger soldiers as they dropped their trousers for injections in both buttocks. The sizable amount of fluid from the immune globulin made it considerably more painful than a typical shot and prompted the occasional "Mama mia" and expletives, followed by a sheepish, "Sorry ma'am." We worked late into the night, monitoring vitals and keeping watch for adverse reactions. Around 1:00 a.m., we crashed on empty patient cots in the ICU tent.

Since the antitoxin injection had never been given in the muscles before, we needed to check on the soldiers around twelve hours after we gave it. So before we left the next day, we trekked across the sand from the CSH to the Battalion Aid Station, a single tent the size of a large teepee with a twelve-foot diameter. Five of us crowded into the tent with a couple of the soldiers at a time. There was little room for seven grown men as we maneuvered around a medical obstacle course—a stretcher, mountains of gauze, and a defibrillator—in a space fit for two. It could have been a scene from *M*A*S*H*, with soldiers dropping their combat trousers so we could examine their behinds. Sand rained down through the gap at the top of the tent and coated everything—including our hair and the soldiers' butts. It was comical in retrospect, but I really wish I had taken a picture for the FDA regulators in their cubicles back home, so they could appreciate the challenges of giving investigational products in a war zone. Fortunately, the soldiers tolerated the antitoxin (and the situation) well. When we finished, we shook off the sand, packed up our papers, and headed to our SUVs.

As our convoy drove back toward Kuwait City, we hit a patch of soupy sand. Behind the wheel Gray Heppner floored it, but this only dug our spinning wheels deeper into what felt like quicksand. The hottest part of the day was approaching. We had no cell phone coverage, and we were too far from Camp Udairi to hike back. The batteries in our GPS had also died. As if on cue, the wind began to blow, stirring up clouds of sand.

I donned a respirator mask, and we got out of the vehicles and started wandering around stupidly, trying to come up with a plan. The sand swirling around us made us nearly invisible. We should have known better because a couple of days earlier a soldier, hidden by airborne grit in a sandstorm, lost one leg and had the other one mangled after being run over by a tanklike armored personnel carrier.

Suddenly, like a desert mirage, a massive tow truck emerged from the khaki fog. I have no idea how the driver knew we were there, but it seemed as if God had sent him. He deftly hooked us up to a cable and pulled us out of the mire, and we were on our way within minutes. Despite the dead GPS, we managed to find our way back to Camp Doha. We celebrated with a trip to the Green Bean, a little white trailer across the base that was the army's answer to Starbucks. A vanilla Frappuccino never tasted so good.

That evening was the first night of shock and awe. Gray Heppner and I climbed up the stairs into the Tactical Operations Center, which was just thirty feet from our office in the headquarters. From the top of a massive amphitheater, we could peer through a large plate-glass window into the room where the bombing campaign was being orchestrated. The three-star general running the operation appeared surprisingly calm, although I suspected he wasn't.

Seeing the attack unfold before me filled me with awe at the numerous individuals functioning as a seamless team. Like a colony of ants quivering in motion, around fifty staffers worked in concert, each with a unique skill: the operations cell, logistics, communication, movement readiness officer, medical evacuation, and air force liaison. Soldiers shuttled back and forth from one cell to another, up and down the stairs like a giant nerve network. The air felt electric. Different colored lights moved in all directions on three-story-high monitors, with each light signifying the movement of our military air attacks. Occasionally the lights flashed, or video feeds showed explosives launched by jets and drones, like a real-life video game.

In the next couple of days, all those forces we had seen driving on the sands toward Udairi launched into Iraq. Casualty counts began to climb. The pace of Scud missile attacks increased. At any time during the day or night, the low-pitched whirring sound of the base siren jolted us to attention. One afternoon, while I was carrying my lunch tray in the dining hall, the siren started to wail. The booming "big voice" on the loudspeaker announced: "TAKE SHELTER. THIS IS NOT A DRILL. MASK NOW." A thousand Velcro flaps ripped open simultaneously as everyone automatically pulled out his or her gas mask. I dropped my tray and fell to the floor.

Another time we were sorting documents in the medical warehouse when the siren sounded. I reached for my mask. It was missing. I cursed myself for accidentally leaving it on my cot. I sat bare-faced breathing into my T-shirt while my colleagues laughed through their masks as they ribbed me with mock eulogies: "We knew him well . . ." I envisioned "drowning under a green sea" with the onset of nerve agent symptoms, like the choking chlorine gas victim in the famous World War I poem, "Dulce et decorum est." I silently prayed for the "ALL CLEAR!" big voice.

One night in the "cave" warehouse, we had repeated alerts, and I had to don and doff my protective suit and mask repeatedly. I awoke in the middle of the night, surprised that I had fallen asleep with my gas mask on. I had grown so comfortable wearing it by then that I no longer felt the horrific claustrophobia.

After we gave the first round of vaccines, we faced a significant dilemma. The botulism vaccine, to be fully effective, requires three closely timed shots—an initial dose, followed by a second dose two weeks later, and a third six weeks after the first. But in that span of time, our soldiers dispersed all over the war zone. Was it worth hitching a ride on a Blackhawk into enemy fire to deliver a few booster shots? Our team leader felt obligated to do it, and we all worried about being chastised for not following through on the prespecified vaccine schedule. It was our duty, after all, to try and protect these soldiers. But dodging mortars in a combat zone to give a booster shot seemed absurd and foolish. Bullethead's elite team was already on the move to undisclosed locations deep inside Iraq. We had no guarantee we could even commandeer a Blackhawk to get to them, much less find them. And the enemy was regularly shooting Blackhawks out of the sky. During one of our team meetings, I protested.

As the junior member, my contrary opinion was dismissed, so I spoke with a more-senior member off-line, who agreed with me. He raised the issue at another meeting. Our leader eventually backed down.

We had to plan our activities not only around missions and battles but also around the local weather, which in Kuwait meant vicious sandstorms. Kuwait's desert sand is a far cry from the grainy, white sand at the Jersey shore. It's more like dried mud pulverized into brown talcum powder. It doesn't take much to get it aloft. After a howling wind, suspended particles would hover in the air while an eerie silence settled over the camp. Everything in sight would be engulfed in airborne silt as thick as pea soup. It was so dense that I nearly turned into a speed bump for a Humvee one evening. By the time I saw the lights penetrating the sand fog, the Hummer was just a few feet away.

Even under clear skies on routine days, it was amazing how important little things mattered at war. An army "runs on its stomach," and we became spoiled by the surprisingly good food. In addition to regular servings of burgers, baked beans, and steak, every lunch and dinner ended with a slice of pie, rotating from apple to cherry to pumpkin. One day the pie disappeared. No warning, no explanation. The replacement was a dry strawberry sponge cake.

"This is highly irregular," we concluded. "Someone has to do something."

Our two senior colonels weren't taking this affront lying down. They marched into the kitchen and backed the sergeant first class in charge up against the wall. "Sergeant, what has happened to the pie? Do you realize what an important morale issue this is for the soldiers? We need our pie!" "Yes . . . yes, sirs," the sergeant responded. "I'll go see if I can find some more pie in the freezers."

The next day the pie returned. We celebrated with an extra helping.

At this point, even with bullets and bombs flying, we still had one more set of hospital staff to train. One sunny morning five of us hopped on a Blackhawk for a ride to the *Comfort,* the navy's hospital ship cruising in the Arabian Gulf. It was exhilarating lifting off from Camp Doha over the sea of tan warehouses below. We flew by the radio towers and spires in downtown Kuwait City and watched the desert recede as we headed out over the water.

The twenty-five-minute flight took us over shimmering blue water until a white rectangle appeared in the distance. As we approached, the rectangle grew into a massive white ship with a large red cross on its side. We touched down on the gray and white striped helipad and ducked out while the turning rotors above washed us with wind. The ship's executive officer, dressed in brown khakis, showed us to our quarters where we would bunk for the night—patient beds again, in an empty hospital ward.

We set up our laptops and projectors in one of the ICUs and briefed the staff. Next we had a tour of the ship. Kyle Peterson, a navy infectious disease doc, showed us around the medical ICU and the isolation room. The capabilities on this ship would be the envy of any hospital director—multiple operating rooms, ICUs, an excellent lab, and a massive blood bank. Kyle was the first doc to report antibiotic-resistant *Acinetobacter* during Operation Iraqi Freedom from patients he cared for on this ship. Treating our battle-wounded soldiers infected with this difficult-to-treat bacteria would later prove a significant challenge for me on the wards of Walter Reed Army Medical Center back home.

Once our work was done, we had no way "off the island," so we spent the rest of the afternoon lounging in the sun on a bed of thick rope on the helipad. The fresh sea air and singing gulls were a welcome contrast from the dusty desert. It was the high point of my deployment. I wondered whether I had joined the wrong branch of the military, because the navy docs seemed to have a pretty good deal.

After spending the night and wrapping up training with the medical staff, we had to wait for a ride back to land. Like the old television *M*A*S*H** episodes, at this point in the war, choppers were in high demand, ferrying casualties from the front lines. When we finally heard the familiar *WHOP-WHOP-WHOP* of an incoming Blackhawk, we were ready to go. The Blackhawk touched down, and the rotors slowed but did not stop. Head down and crouching, I lined up behind my team members on the helipad feeling the rotor wash tussle our hats and uniforms. As I prepared to climb aboard, Bob Kuschner turned to me with three awful words. "KORTEPETER!" he yelled over the roar. "YOU'RE STAYING!"

Four seats. Five bodies. Someone had to stay.

Tail tucked, I retreated to the edge of the helipad. As the Black-hawk rose, I blinked into the blast of air, stunned, and watched the helicopter shrink and vanish in the white-hot sky.

I had to fight back the tears. I'm not particularly superstitious, but this sudden separation from my team felt like a terrible omen. I could not shake the feeling that their chopper—or mine—was doomed. One of my colleagues snapped a photo of me from the Blackhawk, standing alone on the tarmac as they left me behind. This was the lowest point of the mission for me, and it shows on my face.

The same Blackhawk that picked up my teammates had deliv-ered a brown body bag. I retreated into the alcove next to the heli-pad as the medical staff carried it in. Before sliding it into a storage refrigerator, a ship doctor unzipped the thick brown plastic to record some information. I caught a glimpse of the marine's pale left hand, labeled with a paper tag.

The sight of that ghostlike, still hand amplified my dark premoni-tion. Sullen, and not knowing when my ride would come, I retreated to the bowels of the ship, where I found a desk at a vacant nurse's station. I found a ballpoint pen and white-lined paper and wrote an angry and sad letter to my wife, thinking it might be my last.

Soon enough a chopper came for me. Fortunately, I made it back to Camp Doha to reunite with my team and made a celebratory visit to the Green Bean for a latte.

After two months, teams searching for Saddam's cache of biologi-cal and chemical weapons had come up dry. Perhaps Saddam's army had destroyed them after all. Our team was no longer needed. It was time to go home.

I felt satisfied that we had accomplished what we were sent to do, and we did it in a timely fashion. Despite the blinding sand-storms, incoming Scuds, and regulatory nightmares, we had suc-cessfully deployed vaccines and treatments in the theater of war to protect the forces. But opinions of the team members varied. One said, "We were sent on a fool's mission" with an impossible task and outdated vaccines and treatments. We were lucky, after all. The U.S. forces advanced without being attacked with chemical or bio-logical weapons. We were prepared to treat botulism casualties in a small military unit; however, orchestrating a massive botulinum anti-toxin response would have faced formidable challenges. We probably would have failed, at least in meeting all the FDA requirements. No doubt, we would have taken some of the blame.

Defending against bio agents on the battlefield remains a significant challenge. Because their use against our forces would likely be covert, we wouldn't know we had been infected until soldiers became ill in droves. That would be too late. We need licensed countermeasures, but knowing which agent the adversary might reach for is a crapshoot. Research and development efforts continue, but it is unlikely we would ever create vaccines and treatments against all potential threats. If we are successful in licensing one countermeasure, our adversary may just reach for a different agent.

Some of our vulnerabilities from this deployment remain. A new, licensed botulism vaccine is years away. I would like to say that the next effort might be different, but I can't. We would be reinventing the same wheel. Whoever does this before the next war would run up against the same regulatory challenges and mountains of paperwork that we faced. Institutional memories are short, and my colleagues and I who gained experience from this deployment have all moved on. The military still does not get any wider latitude for operational use than any civilian agency. Developing new countermeasures takes years, potentially decades, and there is no easy workaround. There is one bit of good news, though: we now have two licensed botulism antitoxins for the nation, which were first developed at USAMRIID.

I had mixed emotions about leaving the desert. I had really enjoyed the camaraderie with my teammates and knew I could never replicate the action and excitement of the deployment. My original concerns about being out of my league with my more-senior colleagues had long since abated, and we had become friends. However, I did not look forward to returning to the usual leadership frustrations back at USAMRIID, and my guilt over lacking enthusiasm about having another child also returned.

Landing at Dulles International Airport in Washington DC was bittersweet. I just picked up my duffle bags from baggage claim and said a quick goodbye to my teammates. At one moment we were a close-knit team operating on the fringe of the world, and in the next we went our separate ways. I took a quiet, lonely cab ride home.

Seeing my family brightened my spirits, though. Sean had made a card that said, "Welcome Home Daddy" in black marker. On the inside of the card, he wrote, "I can do my . . ." followed by a page of his alphabets, in different sizes and shapes in red marker. Luke wanted to show me he had a haircut. He drew pictures of "me before" and "me after," where the first one looked normal and the second one frazzled with much shorter hair. Inside he wrote: "We are glad your back. At baseball I got hit by the pitch. Everyone is glad you came back." Cindy had enlisted ten-year-old Luke to serve as her birth "coach" in case I didn't make it back.

The next morning Cindy and I walked out to the front lawn with the boys. She handed me a pair of scissors to cut the yellow ribbon she had tied around the cherry tree in front of our house.

Ten days later whatever concerns I had about becoming a father again melted away as I held the squirming nine-pound, three-ounce gift as he entered the world. I enjoyed holding this little bundle against my chest as we both fell asleep each night. To this day he has the most infectious smile, and I am grateful for fatherhood each day.

13

Desert Pneumonia

....

After returning from the desert in May 2003, I resumed my prior job as chief of the Medical Division at USAMRIID. By then U.S. forces had advanced throughout Iraq. I had some difficulty refocusing at first on the daily minutiae of administration after dealing with the more serious life-or-death issues in the desert. I almost welcomed a new challenge that awakened me from my postdeployment doldrums.

Sometimes I found myself serving as a nexus or a tripwire for responding to or sounding the alarm about infectious disease crises elsewhere in the military. There had been occasional reports of pneumonia among troops deployed to the Middle East for the war. In March 2003 there had been some email chatter when two severely ill soldiers were treated for pneumonia at the Landstuhl Regional Medical Center in Germany after being evacuated from Iraq. These cases were deemed to be the normal background disease incidence. Not an outbreak.

On June 17, 2003, a soldier with severe pneumonia was in the process of being evacuated from Iraq to Germany, but he died before leaving the country.

Around this time, the air force transferred a new infectious disease physician to work in my division. Lieutenant Colonel Janice Rusnak was a quiet, medium-height blonde who loved horses.

The air force had a position for an infectious disease doctor at the Landstuhl Regional Medical Center in Germany, the first stop for ill and wounded soldiers and marines evacuated from Afghanistan and Iraq. In the summer of 2003, when the physician rotated out of Landstuhl for his next assignment, the air force tagged Janice to cover for a couple of months until a replacement arrived.

In late June we at USAMRIID had some dialogue with personnel at the Twenty-Eighth Combat Support Hospital in Iraq about a severely ill soldier they were caring for with pneumonia. In an update email I received on June 26 from a doctor at the CSH, he wrote, "He [the ill soldier] will be leaving tonight to Germany." A picture of the patient's chest X-ray was attached to the email.

While she was in Germany, Janice usually received advanced warning of incoming infectious disease–related air evacuations, but I sent her a heads-up email anyway: "Looks like he may be on his way to you shortly." The chest X-ray looked bad, with a whiteout of both lungs, so I copied Colonel (Dr.) Tim Endy, my fellow USAMRIID division chief in Virology. He forwarded my email on to some of his infectious disease colleagues in case they had ideas about possible causes. For the same reason, I also sent the note to my USAMRIID colleagues, writing "Impressive CXR [chest X-ray] findings."

The soldier arrived in Landstuhl, and Janice was asked to evaluate him. Janice rode the elevator to the ICU, where the patient was being cared for. She got out and turned left toward the ICU, which had a long central corridor, with an open bay on the left and single-patient rooms on the right. When she entered the ICU, she asked the nurse where the soldier with pneumonia on a ventilator, recently evacuated from Iraq, was located.

"Which one?" the nurse responded. "We have three."[1]

Whoa! Janice thought immediately, feeling like her stomach had jumped up into her throat. Three young soldiers requiring ventilators at the same time? Janice evaluated the patient she was asked to see and wrote up her recommendations, but she was particularly concerned because this patient was the third case of severe pneumonia in the past month from the same CSH in Iraq. One of those prior cases was the soldier who had died a mere ten days earlier. Now there were two additional cases on ventilators from Iraq? Janice wanted to know what might be causing such a severe illness in young, healthy soldiers.

On June 30 Janice copied Tim Endy and me on an email she sent to doctors in Iraq describing the situation: "There are currently three young (ages 20–22 years) AD [active duty] intubated with ARDS [acute respiratory distress syndrome] in the ICU."

Tagged onto that note was an earlier one written by someone at the CSH in Iraq: "We have another patient that just arrived today with the same clinical findings. . . . We're getting pretty anxious now suspecting a trend."

Janice alerted the chiefs of Pulmonology and of Medicine at Landstuhl about the possibility of an outbreak. She started to review charts of pneumonia cases that had come through Landstuhl from Iraq during the prior six months. She also put together a panel of labs for testing on anyone with "Iraq pneumonia."

Back at USAMRIID, we were hearing rumors of seventeen other pneumonia patients.

This scared me. It could be nothing. We always hope it is. But it could also be a disaster. Was I hearing the hoofbeats of zebras?

Three things make up the "epidemiologic triangle," and all three must align to start an outbreak: a pathogen, a host (like a human) infected by the pathogen, and an environment that facilitates spread. The third factor is the most important for triggering the chain reaction for an outbreak. Ebola might kill an occasional, undiagnosed victim in the jungle, but move that victim to a hospital, and the epidemiologic triangle forms, causing the disease to explode.

I worried that the epi-triangle pieces had aligned. Something lurking in the desert was facilitating spread. Janice's cases could be the sentinel for a bigger disaster on the way.

I wasn't the only one thinking along those lines.

A few minutes after receiving Janice's email, my phone rang, with Tim Endy on the line. He was in the middle of his month-long rotation as the consulting infectious disease physician at Walter Reed Army Medical Center. "Mark," he said, "We're following a woman in the ICU with the same thing." She had also been medically evacuated from Iraq.

Shit!

I felt that familiar queasiness of impending doom in the pit of my stomach. This could be real. I set the phone down and considered the possibilities. The Severe Acute Respiratory Syndrome (SARS) virus had circled the globe mere months previously. Was SARS staging a comeback? SARS could spell disaster for our battlefield forces. Also, in 1992 Saudi Arabian physicians described a "new clinicopathological entity, Desert Storm pneumonitis or Al Eskan disease . . . when the mixture of fine Saudi dust and pigeon droppings triggered a hyperergic [allergic] lung condition."[2] Could this be Al Eskan or another new disease? Even more worrisome: could this be the Iraqi biological weapon attack that we all feared?

The army pulled our SMART-IND team out of the desert because the risk for bioweapon attack had abated. Was that a mistake?

I could not sit on this.

With my public health background and USAMRIID position I bridged the Army's public health and infectious disease communities. I fired off an email to two leaders: Colonel Bob Defraites, the lead preventive medicine physician at the army surgeon general's office and Dr. Bruno Petruccelli at the Army Center for Health Promotion.

"Bruno and Bob: . . . Some of these cases are particularly concerning and unusual in their severity and rapidity of onset. . . . I'm thinking an EPICON [epidemiologic consultation] investigation might be useful. What do you think?"

I followed up immediately with a phone call. "Bob, Mark Kortepeter here. I think we have a problem. Look at the email I just forwarded to you."

Bob set up a call for a small group to confer and decide how to respond.

The first thing you do in a cardiac arrest in the hospital is take your own pulse. For an outbreak investigation, we first take a step back and tease fact apart from rumor to decide whether there really is an outbreak. Then we try to make a diagnosis and determine how many patients really have the problem and whether it is the same problem. Next decide whether the disease frequency is different from the norm and who might be at risk.

Word spread quickly, and the vast military infectious disease and preventive medicine network began to mobilize. Doctors in-country told us that soldiers had numerous exposures to rodents, mosquitoes, sandflies, fleas, and ticks, which raised lots of possibilities for infections. Dr. Charles Hoke, former consultant to the surgeon general for infectious diseases offered several potential diagnoses—"tularemia, plague, typhus, malaria, hantavirus pulmonary syndrome, SARS"—but in the desert, they had no ability to get bacterial cultures, do Gram stains, or get antibody testing, and the choice of antibiotics was limited. By the time the soldiers arrived in Germany, any antibiotics they might have received already made it too late to pick up the offending organisms with a bacterial culture. We were flying blind.

We had a teleconference the next day to do what any public health team would do at the start of an outbreak: describe the disease, develop a case definition, and generate a differential diagnosis.

We came up with a case definition:

> Onset of illness in a deployed service member since 1 March while stationed in Iraq or Kuwait with:
>
> 1) any radiographic sign of pneumonitis or pneumonia OR
>
> 2) severe respiratory distress requiring intubation OR
>
> 3) sudden unexplained death

Armed with this case definition, Bob's team at the surgeon general's office conducted a preliminary review of the surveillance data. Approximately one hundred personnel had been treated for pneumonia. Among those, fourteen soldiers and one marine had developed severe pneumonia that required medical evacuation to Landstuhl. There appeared to be no geographic link.

Preliminary lab data came up negative for a cause, even from an autopsy conducted on the June 17 death. Labs were forwarded to Landstuhl and to USAMRIID for additional testing.

The lead medical general in-theater emailed the growing list of addresses on the email string, currently at nine, "I am in favor of an EPICON/EPIAID [epidemiologic consultation]. . . . I am concerned that something is going on here, although on the surface we cannot find any patterns." In two days the email list would grow to thirty-two, a week later to sixty-three, as the urgency increased, and the network expanded.

We all had similar concerns. During our initial telephone conference, we discussed the possibility of launching an investigative team. In the next week, sentiments for a team shifted back and forth. Numerous docs weighed in on potential causes, and some disagreed

whether this was pneumonia or pulmonary edema. More information rolled in about possible exposures after an interview with a
victim, which expanded the list of potential diagnoses: "The buildings they stay in were filled with three feet of trash including feces
of both human and animals. There are pigeons all over the place-
like you would not believe. They sleep outside because it is too hot
to sleep in the 'cleaned' building . . . loads of mosquito bites . . . dead
cats and dogs, few dead horses, few dead people in the streets. He
routinely patrols through knee high sewage."

The environment was an infectious disease doctor's nightmare.

On July 12 the next shoe dropped. A second soldier died.

No more time to wait. Bruno Petruccelli sent out an urgent note
in advance of a scheduled telephone conference on July 16: "Please
remove the word 'standby' [for the team]. . . . It's now ASAP to deploy."

Four days later, the first investigative team launched to Germany.

On August 1 the news hit *Promed*, the online outbreak alert notification system: "Army sends team to probe Iraq Illness."

The second team shipped out August 5 for Iraq.

An average of 183,000 military personnel had moved through Iraq
during this period. The teams sent to Germany and Iraq had to tease
apart the potential for a natural versus an engineered attack. They
sorted through patient records, lab results, radiographic results, and
interviewed staff and patients looking for clues. They administered
questionnaires covering a battery of possible risks: tobacco use,
vaccines received, sleeping locations, contact with prisoners, water
sources, use of medications, insect repellents, contacts with chemicals, illicit drugs. Team members collected samples of tobacco products for testing for contamination with paraquat, bacteria, fungi, and
specific threats like ricin, strychnine, and other toxins.[3]

After months of work, including a myriad of laboratory tests, the
investigation of desert pneumonia discovered that nineteen soldiers
who had deployed to Iraq and surrounding countries had developed
severe pneumonia and required a ventilator to survive. Two died.
The peak occurred in June and July, which was why they hit our radar
screen then. Several had been infected with common bacteria like

pneumococcus. Strangely, ten had elevated levels of eosinophils, a white blood cell that spikes with allergies or parasite infections. In those patients antibiotics didn't work. Even before the epidemiology investigation had concluded, the Medical Division chief and one of the pulmonary doctors at Landstuhl elected to treat some soldiers who had elevated eosinophils or wheezing with steroids, and it seemed to help.

The only common risk identified among the ill was smoking. Fourteen of them had begun smoking after deploying. Could another exposure on top of the cigarettes and desert dust have led to the pneumonia, as in the case of Al Eskan disease years earlier? We never determined conclusively why so many had gotten sick and why then.

Even so the good news was that this wasn't a bioweapon attack, but we were right to be concerned. When I first read Janice's emails about soldiers with pneumonia, my experience and position gave me the confidence and authority to pick up the phone and reach out to my public health contacts to kick-start an investigation. We could then leverage the infectious disease and preventive medicine communities and the sophisticated lab testing available through the military's lab network. Everyone came together to run this to ground.

Having the ability to respond rapidly works for natural disease outbreaks like pneumonia in the desert as well as our next disaster brewing over the horizon in an African country most people have probably never heard of.

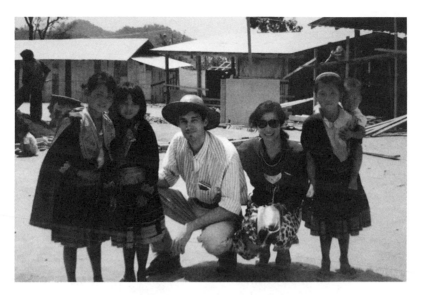

1. The author with his wife, Cindy, while attending a tropical medicine meeting in Thailand, 1991. My training in Hawaii inspired a lifelong interest in infectious diseases and tropical medicine. From the author's collection.

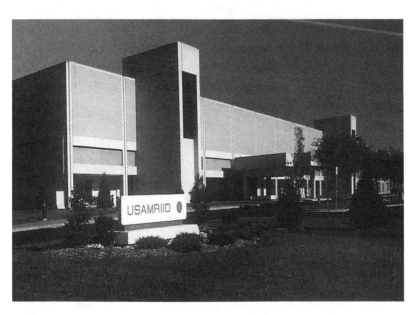

2. The U.S. Army Medical Research Institute of Infectious Diseases (USAMRIID), Fort Detrick, Maryland. Courtesy of Caree Vander Linden and USAMRIID.

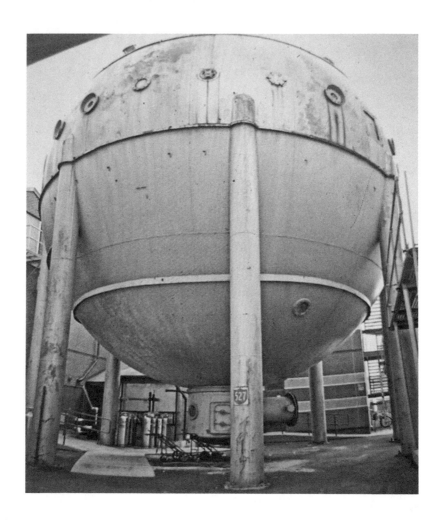

3. The 8 Ball at Fort Detrick, a one-million-liter sphere used to do aerosol exposure testing on humans and animals for biothreat agents and vaccine testing. Courtesy of USAMRIID.

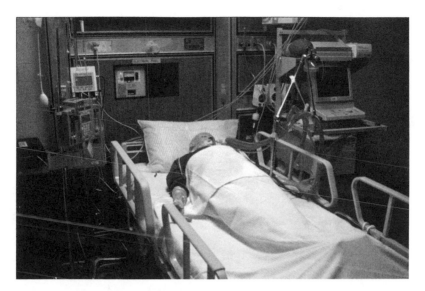

4. The "Slammer" isolation facility inside USAMRIID, where patients with lab or field exposures to infectious biothreat agents might be monitored for illness or cared for once ill. Courtesy of Rick Stevens and USAMRIID

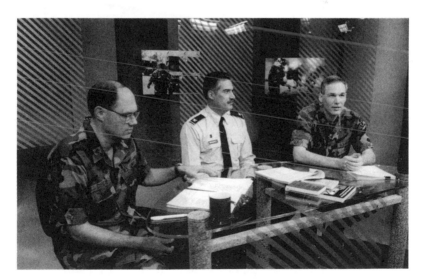

5. The author on camera with colleagues Ted Cieslak (left) and Toti Sanchez (center) during an award-winning live satellite television broadcast "Biowarfare and Terrorism, the Military and Public Health Response," 1999. Courtesy of Barbara Richards and FDA studios, Gaithersburg, Maryland.

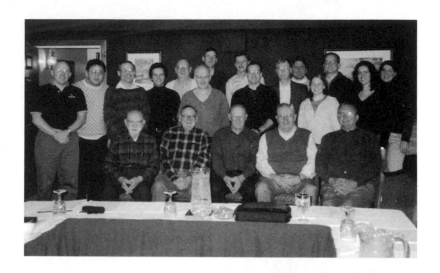

6. With senior biodefense leaders at a biothreat meeting, St. Michaels, Maryland, ca. 1999. Left to right, front row: Abram Benenson, Bill Patrick, Phil Russell, DA Henderson, Charles Bailey; second row: John Wade, Ken Alibek, Ted Hadfield, Steven Becker, Tom Monath, unknown, Peter Jahrling, unknown, unknown; third row: David Huxholl, Mark Kortepeter, David Franz, Les Caudal, David Ashford, unknown. From the author's collection, courtesy of David Franz.

7. (*opposite top*) In my office at USAMRIID when I was the chief of the Medical Division, ca. 2001. Courtesy of Denise Clizbe.

8. (*opposite bottom*) John Ezzell, chief of the USAMRIID Special Pathogens Lab showing the Daschle anthrax letter from inside the BSL-3 lab, 2001. Courtesy of John Ezzell and USAMRIID.

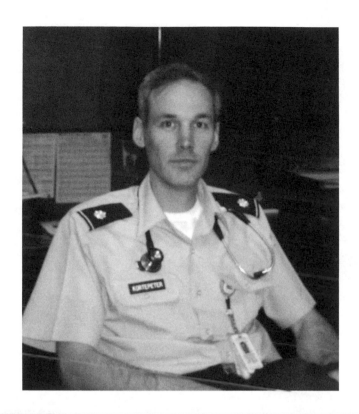

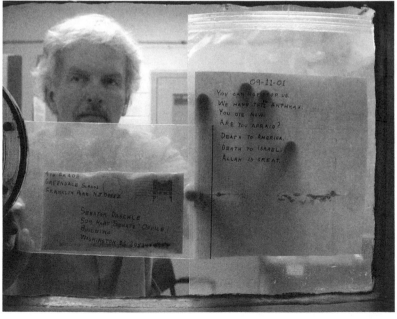

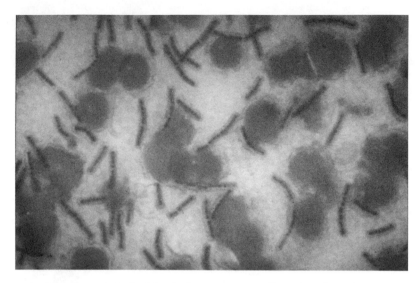

9. Anthrax bacteria in the blood of an experimentally infected monkey. Courtesy of USAMRIID.

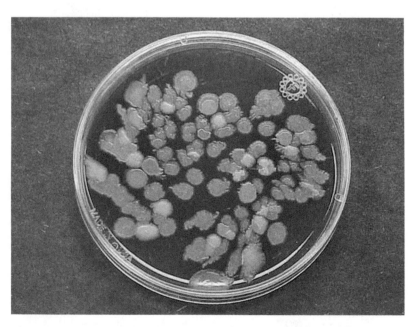

10. Petri dish showing colony shade and shape variants of *Bacillus anthracis* (causative agent of anthrax). Courtesy of Pat Worsham and USAMRIID.

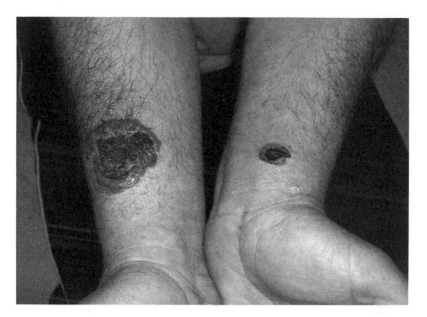

11. A shepherd with cutaneous anthrax after slaughtering a sheep, seen by the author, Rob Rivard, and Michael Ellis in Tbilisi, Republic of Georgia. The patient received intramuscular penicillin for three days, so the swelling had improved, but he still had the black eschars typically seen with anthrax. Courtesy of Robert Rivard.

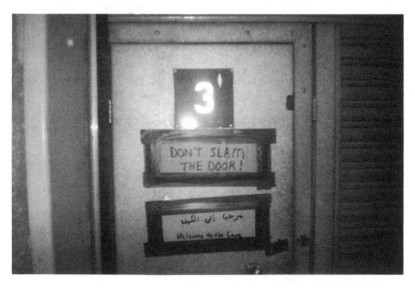

12. The entrance to the "Cave" warehouse, where the author slept on a cot, Camp Doha, Kuwait, 2003. From the author's collection.

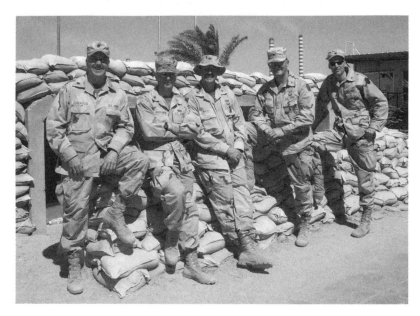

13. Doctors on the SMART-IND team in front of a bunker for Scud missile attacks, Camp Doha, Kuwait, 2003. Left to right: Chris Ockenhouse, Robert Kuschner, Alan Magill, Gray Hepper, Mark Kortepeter. From the author's collection.

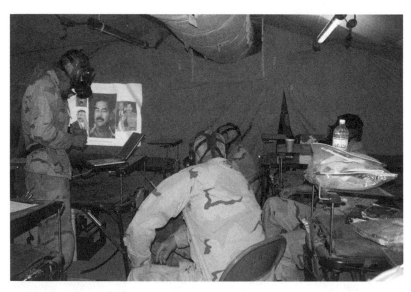

14. The author giving a biothreat briefing in the middle of a Scud missile attack to physicians at the Twenty-Eighth Combat Support Hospital, Camp Udairi, Kuwait, 2003. Courtesy of Coleen Martinez.

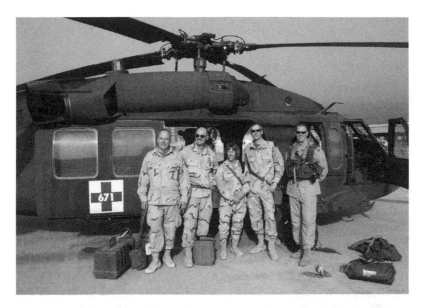

15. SMART-IND team members en route to provide training on biowarfare countermeasures on the *Comfort* hospital ship, Camp Doha, Kuwait, 2003. Left to right: Chris Ockenhouse, Alan Magill, Jackie Carlin, Mark Kortepeter, unknown pilot. Courtesy of Robert Kuschner.

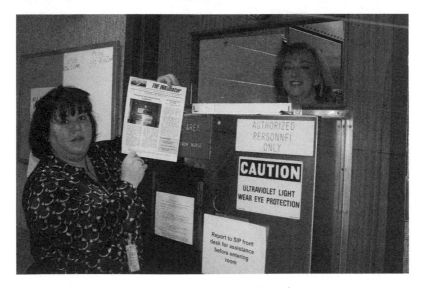

16. Denise Clizbe (outside) and Kelly Warfield (inside) the Slammer. Kelly's delight upon being released on this date from the Slammer is evident. Denise is holding a mock newsletter titled "Prisoner Released from the Slammer." Courtesy of Denise Clizbe and Kelly Warfield.

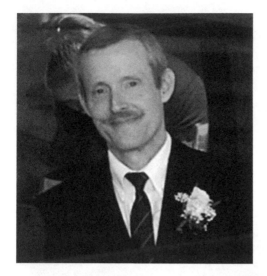

17. Bruce Ivins, bacteriologist at USAMRIID at an awards ceremony in 2003. Ivins was named by the FBI as the perpetrator of the 2001 anthrax letters but committed suicide prior to a trial. After his death this photo was provided to the press after consideration by the author and the USAMRIID Public Affairs Officer. Courtesy of USAMRIID.

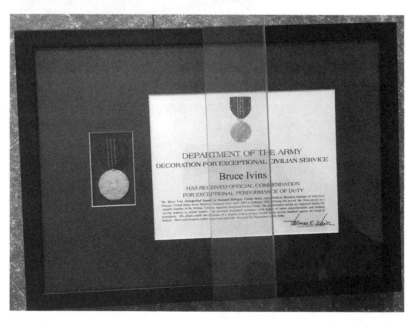

18. "Decoration for Exceptional Civilian Service" award given to Bruce Ivins for service to the government, Bacteriology Division, USAMRIID. Courtesy of Caree Vander Linden and USAMRIID.

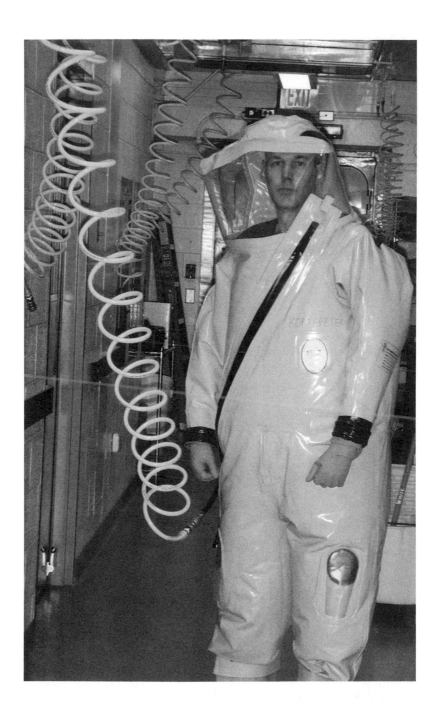

19. The author inside the BSL-4 lab, AA-4, at USAMRIID when conducting a nonhuman primate study of Ebola, 2009. Courtesy of Gene Olinger.

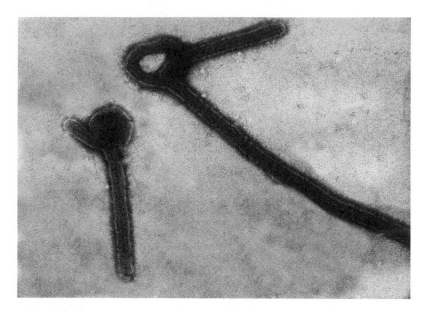

20. An electron micrograph of Ebola virus demonstrating its long, spindly shape. Magnification 80,000X. Courtesy of Xiankun (Kevin) Zeng and USAMRIID.

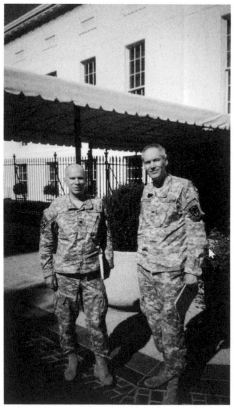

21. The author with Robert Rivard outside the West Wing of the White House after providing lectures on biodefense to the White House medical staff, ca. 2011. Courtesy of Robert Rivard.

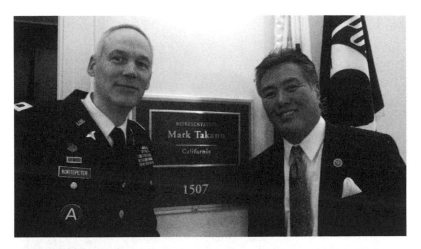

22. The author with California congressman Mark Takano after briefing him on the Ebola outbreak in West Africa, 2014. From the author's collection.

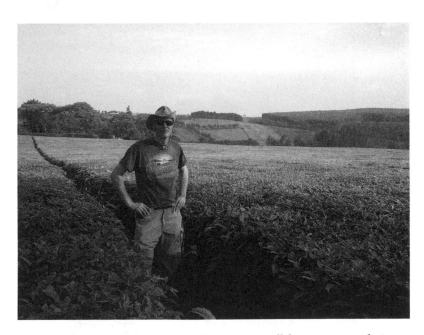

23. The author at a tea plantation while visiting a collaborative research site, Kericho, Kenya, 2013. Courtesy of David Tribble.

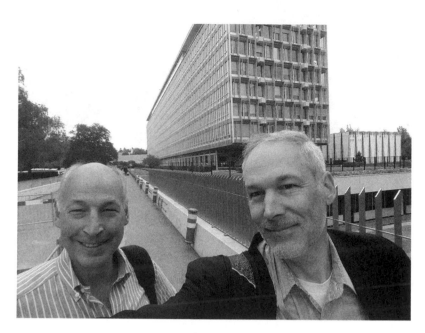

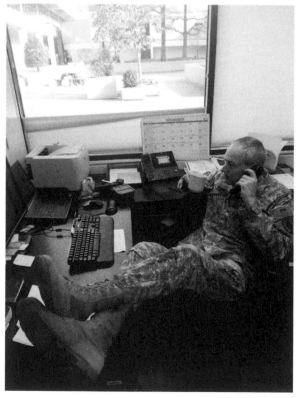

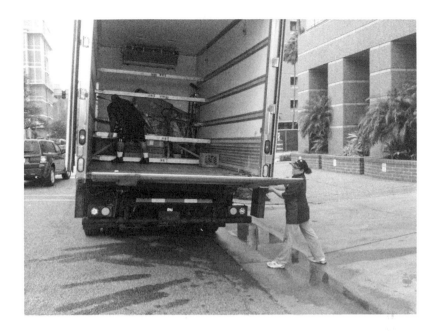

24. (*opposite top*) The author with Simon Mardel, Ebola expert from the United Kingdom, outside the WHO headquarters, Geneva, Switzerland, 2018. From the author's collection.

25. (*opposite bottom*) In my office as the associate dean for research at the Hébert School of Medicine, Uniformed Services University, 2015. Courtesy of Leody Bojanowski.

26. (*above*) The cost of shipping a single freezer box (shown here) with four samples of Marburg virus, each containing 0.25 ml from USAMRIID to the University of Texas, Galveston, was $4,832.87 in 2014. Courtesy of Tom Ksiazek and the University of Texas Medical Branch, Galveston.

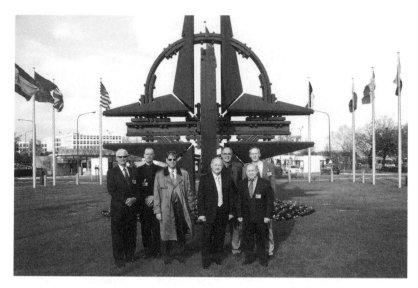

27. With colleagues from the NATO Biomedical Advisory Panel at NATO headquarters, Brussels. Left to right: Tom Bosey, Robert von Tersch, unknown, James Smith, Ted Cieslak, Mark Bohanan, Mark Kortepeter. From the author's collection, courtesy of Ted Cieslak.

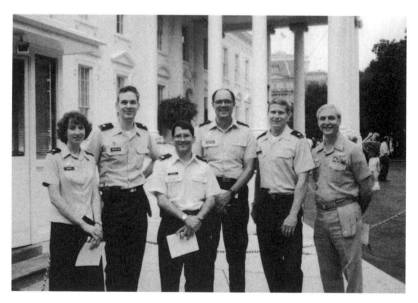

28. USAMRIID operational medicine colleagues at the White House after meeting with White House physician Rob Darling. Left to right: Julie Pavlin, Mark Kortepeter, George Christopher, Ted Cieslak, John Rowe, Randy Culpepper. Courtesy of Rob Darling.

4

The 4M Disaster

Good doctors are of no use without good discipline.

—Lieutenant General William Slim, British Corps commander, Burma, WWII

Even before the ink was dry on the desert pneumonia investigation report, we faced another crisis that pulled USAMRIID and the military infectious disease community together again.

In 2003, long before Ebola struck West Africa, a civil war raged in Liberia. The U.S. military launched the USS *Iwo Jima* Amphibious Ready Group to secure the Roberts International Airport outside Monrovia. The Twenty-Sixth Marine Expeditionary Unit on board arrived from recent deployments to Iraq and Djibouti. Before leaving the ship, each marine received aluminum-wrapped blister packs of mefloquine pills to take weekly on the honor system to prevent malaria. They also received the standard briefing on guarding themselves against mosquito bites: sleep under bed nets, spray your uniforms with the insecticide permethrin, and use insect repellents.

On August 14, 2003, nine helicopters took off from the ship's deck and ferried 225 marines ashore. The marines set up their living quarters inside an abandoned, rat-infested airport warehouse surrounded by broken windows, standing water, and swarms of mosquitoes. The marines cleaned out the debris and swept the site to make it more hospitable, and some hung out on the roof. Anyone who knows anything about military history might have predicted the impending fiasco.

The marines spent a mere eleven days on the ground before returning to their ships. After one day back on the ship, a marine spiked a fever. Others with fever and diarrhea soon followed. Shipboard doctors gave them the antibiotic ciprofloxacin to treat presumed travelers' diarrhea. Thus began the disaster.

Liberia happens to be a hot spot for Lassa fever, a deadly virus that causes a hemorrhagic fever like Ebola, but it is easier to catch. The discovery of Lassa fever in 1969 occurred after an incredible convergence of events and bad luck. Laura Wine, a nurse at the Lassa Mission Hospital in Nigeria, probably cared for an unrecognized victim before she developed a fever with severe fatigue, back pain, sore throat, and rash. Seven days later her kidneys shut down, her face swelled, she convulsed, and then she died. Charlotte Shaw, a fellow mission nurse, contaminated a cut on her finger with Laura's saliva while caring for her. She soon came down with a 102-degree fever, headache, chills, and back and leg pains. Malaria pills didn't help. Within eleven days Charlotte's blood pressure plummeted, she swelled, and she also died. Penny Pinneo, a third nurse who cared for both Wine and Shaw, developed a low-grade fever, weakness, and dizziness. The mission doctors, recognizing a disturbing chain of transmission and afraid Penny might die, too, flew her emergently to the United States for treatment. After several grueling days of travel, she finally arrived for care at Columbia Presbyterian Hospital in New York City. Miraculously, she survived. The hospital doctors worked closely with the virology laboratory at Yale, which had received blood samples from all three nurses. After painstaking work over months collaborating with the CDC, they discovered a new virus, named Lassa after the Nigerian town of its first victims.

Field studies revealed that Lassa survives in West African rats that shed large amounts of virus in their urine and feces. Humans are infected in multiple ways: after eating food contaminated with rat urine or feces, eating the rats (a delicacy in parts of West Africa), or inhaling the virus in an enclosed area.

On Friday, September 5, an ocean away from Liberia, USAMRIID held a badly needed "morale day" for institute personnel, which included a raft expedition down the Shenandoah River in West Virginia. My clinic chief, Dr. Ellen Boudreau, decided to forgo the event and work instead, because she feared recent heavy rains might increase the risk of hazardous rapids. I had the opposite view, hoping the rains guaranteed extra excitement on the rapids.

Ellen spent a quiet morning catching up on her research paperwork back at USAMRIID. Around 3:30 p.m., USAMRIID's headquarters patched in a call to her office from an air force major, the military flight dispatcher in Germany.

"How did you get my name?" Ellen asked. "They told me you would know something, and you were the best person around at the time," the dispatcher said. "What can I help you with?" Ellen responded.

The dispatcher described a nightmarish scenario, with marines sleeping in a rat-infested warehouse. Now some were sick, and he had the two sickest loaded on a plane on the tarmac at the Monrovia, Liberia, airport. They thought it might be Lassa fever. Should he send them to USAMRIID?

Ellen pulled in colleague Dr. John Aldis, and the two of them engaged with the dispatcher in a series of phone calls that got their undivided attention. They couldn't talk to anyone on the ship directly, but they relayed questions and answers through the dispatcher to the ship.

John is a family-practice doctor with a Tulane public health degree who spent ten years in the navy and then eighteen years as a U.S. embassy physician in the foreign service in places like Indonesia, the Philippines, and West Africa before coming to USAMRIID. His gray hair and wire-framed glasses give him a scholarly appearance.

"We were first trying to figure out what the fuck was going on," John said. "I pictured in my mind five or six marines and two or three were extremely ill." A couple of marines "were essentially dying. That news came through pretty quickly early on. Extremely sick marines" who were becoming "less and less responsive, less and less coherent."

There was no one else around USAMRIID at the time to consult with. "The place was basically deserted," John said. "We felt a bit lonely. This was Friday afternoon. Nobody was home. Nobody was answering phones. Nobody was helping us. It was unbelievable. Both of us slipped into our 'tropical medicine' mode and started with some questions. . . . Anyone with severe fever coming out of that area would have malaria until proven otherwise."

Malaria, a known tropical scourge of military forces for centuries, gets its name from the Latin term for "bad air" because infections occurred around swamps, where the air smelled bad. But it wasn't the air; it was the mosquitoes spreading the deadly parasite.

When female mosquitoes bite someone infected with malaria, the mosquito ingests male and female parasite forms that unite in the mosquito's gut. After two weeks their offspring migrate to the mosquito's salivary glands and the next unlucky person bitten gets injected with thousands of infectious parasites. The parasites travel to the liver and later escape into the blood stream. Like any parasite, they seek nourishment and devour hemoglobin, the molecule in red blood cells that carries oxygen in the bloodstream. After developing inside the cells for a couple of days, the parasites burst out, popping the red cell like a balloon, and seek new red cells to infect. This continues in waves of illness, causing patients to go through cycles of fever and shakes on successive days in synchrony with the parasite's life cycle. Severely ill victims can go into renal failure, respiratory failure, or become unconscious before they die.

"Are they on malaria prophylaxis?" John and Ellen asked the dispatcher. "Yes, yes," was the response. "Are we sure they're taking it?" John asked, and Ellen nodded in agreement with his question. "Oh yes, direct observed therapy," the dispatcher responded. "The sergeant was watching them take it."

John had some skepticism from his own experience with marines. When his brother visited a clinic in Pleku, during the Vietnam War, he was amused to see numerous chloroquine pills, given to prevent malaria, scattered on the ground outside the clinic. "It looked like snow," he said. The marines were "putting pills in their mouths and spitting them out when they got out of the clinic."

Ellen thought, if they had Lassa, the Slammer at USAMRIID might be the best place for them. It was the only unit of its kind in the United States at the time, and its unique features could prevent spread of contagion in the hospital. But Liberia was at least eight hours away. The patients could go downhill fast during the flight and arrive at our doorstep circling the drain. Ellen recommended instead that the dispatcher send the two marines to Landstuhl Regional Medical Center, the closer military hospital in Germany.

Then the dispatcher said that the ship's doctor, a general surgeon, "thinks on the blood smear he sees malarial parasites."

"That just blew us away," John said. "So, then everything shifted. The world turned upside down." John's voice quivers with emotion as he recalls what that meant: "We gotta save these lives and we can do it. Lassa, not much chance. We have to get them in treatment very, very soon. We can't wait on a flight."

He and Ellen insisted: "If they were put on a plane, they must be on treatment. Our feeling was if it was Lassa, starting them on malaria treatment wasn't going to hurt them."

But they got resistance. "Was it really necessary?" the flight dispatcher asked. He wondered why malaria was being considered if the soldiers had indeed been taking their prophylaxis.

John said, "He was a nice guy, but he was as terrified as the rest of us." The dispatcher was worried about a very narrow flight window. "You know," John says, "you don't fight flight windows."

The dispatcher had another problem. "I have a bunch of sick marines on board a ship off the coast of Liberia," he said, "and they want me to take them to get care in the United States for their fevers. They feel that USAMRIID is supposed to be the place to take them. Are you a specialist in this area?"

"It could be several possibilities," Ellen said, "but I'll let you talk to the infectious disease doctor." It just so happened, that doctor was her husband, Colonel Charles Hoke, who by now had retired from the army but who still worked for the army across the street from USAMRIID.

She hung up the phone and contacted Charles immediately. She gave him a brief rundown. Charles looked at his watch, and said, "Oh my gosh, it's 4:30 on a Friday afternoon. Nobody's going to be in the office" at the navy hospital in Bethesda, Maryland.

Charles called the dispatcher back. The dispatcher told him, "Don't take a long time," in a rude and pressured voice. "We've got a big problem. We've got to hurry. We need a decision here. You're holding up a plane."

While on the phone with the dispatcher, Charles thought—*it's an hour earlier in San Antonio, Texas*, home of the Brooke Army Medical Center. He called the infectious disease consultant to the army surgeon general who worked at Brooke and kick-started the extensive military infectious disease network. But these were marines—they should go to a navy hospital instead. With Charles still on the phone, the doctor at Brooke immediately contacted his navy counterpart, Dr. (Captain) Sybil Tasker, on another line.

Sybil notified her hospital chain of command and her team at the National Naval Medical Center (NNMC) in Bethesda, Maryland, to prepare for admitting up to thirty sick marines.

When Charles got off the phone, he called the dispatcher back to let him know that the navy hospital was ramping up. The plane with the two sickest marines had just lifted off en route to Germany.

At the Landstuhl Regional Medical Center in Germany, Lieutenant Colonel Greg Deye, the new infectious disease doctor, got a call about two sick marines who were inbound. As many as thirty to forty might arrive on a later flight.

Oh Shit, he thought.

Greg had little time to prepare, but he spent much of that time fielding calls from generals wanting to hear the latest.

The extremely high attack rate didn't jibe with malaria, especially for marines taking malaria pills. It had the classic hallmarks of a point-source outbreak from a common exposure—like when a whole church congregation develops fever and vomiting after eating the same tainted potato salad at a church picnic. Sybil Tasker worried about Lassa, with rat urine and feces in the warehouse as the common exposure.

One of Sybil's colleagues at NNMC, Dr. (Captain) Greg Martin, got on speed dial with the surgeon on the ship and kept in close contact over the next twenty-four hours. The surgeon told him he had looked at a blood smear from one of the sick marines and thought he saw malaria parasites. Greg was dubious. After all, most surgeons wouldn't know how to diagnose malaria, and the marines were taking mefloquine pills already.

Diagnosing malaria with a microscope requires two drops of blood smeared and stained on a glass slide and a trained eye to recognize its sinister beauty of signet rings or headphone shapes lit up in a splash of dark red, purple, and blue inside the hockey-puck shaped red blood cells. Some species of malaria develop tiny blue stipples or transform into basket, amoeboid, or oval forms with pointy antennae. But the surgeon had taken the military's tropical medicine class a year earlier, where he learned how to identify malaria. So Dr. Greg Martin recommended treating the febrile marines still on the ship for malaria before they got on the plane, just in case.

Greg Martin then got into a tug of war with the air force, which said it wouldn't risk carrying marines infected with a potentially dangerous agent like Lassa, thus contaminating and knocking a multimillion-dollar plane out of commission afterward. Greg dug in his heals and pushed the argument up the chain of command. There was no way he would leave up to forty sick marines stranded in Liberia or on ships. Greg prevailed.

Hours later, in Germany, just as the first two sick marines arrived, Dr. Greg Deye learned the other planeload of thirty to forty marines would be diverted to Washington. He breathed a sigh of relief.

It had been a beautiful, sunny day, and a good time with my USAM-RIID colleagues on the rapids. Around 5:00 p.m. that afternoon, I was pulling my raft out of the Shenandoah River when my cell phone rang. Ellen Boudreau was on the line, and she briefed me about the impending disaster.

After hearing about the rat-infested warehouse, I said, "Shit, that sounds like Lassa." The marines would have had plenty of opportunities to contact or inhale the virus. We had a stash of the only possible treatment for Lassa, an investigational antiviral drug, ribavirin, so we kept an active protocol for the occasional unlucky soldier or lab worker who might get infected. We hadn't used the ribavirin protocol for several years, so I recommended my team "dust it off," just in case we needed to use it.

Lassa had a track record for spreading in the hospital, but scientists had also learned the hard way that Lassa spreads just as easily inside the laboratory. In 1969 the chief lab scientist at Yale, Dr. Jordi Casals, became severely ill and nearly died. Convalescent serum, donated by Penny Pinneo, may have saved his life. One of his technicians, Juan Ramon, also became ill. Because Ramon had not worked with the virus, no one considered the possibility of Lassa until it was too late. He died. No one knew how Lassa got him, but as a result Dr. Casals moved further research with the virus to the national Communicable Disease Center laboratory (precursor to the CDC) in Atlanta. These events helped shepherd in a new era of studying such dangerous viruses in highly controlled "containment" laboratories at the CDC and USAMRIID.

Mindful of Lassa's checkered history, Sybil Tasker didn't want to raise a panic at NNMC during the weekend, but she had to prepare for the risk of spread within the hospital, just as one would for Ebola virus. If the marines on their way to Washington had Lassa, she considered the major cluster it would be to care for them safely, feed them, and set up guards for the ward. The team at NNMC moved boatloads of patients to empty out an entire thirty-four-bed cancer ward to isolate the ill marines.

A brand-new infectious disease fellow-in-training was in the doctors' room at NNMC and thought he overhead one of the staff say there was a plane of inbound marines sick with "Wassa fever." Not knowing what that was, he immediately looked it up online. The internet response, "Do you mean Lassa fever?" Oh, *Lassa* fever.

As the night wore on and the navy doctors went through their preparation checklists, they considered that if the marines on the hospital wards used the toilets, they could potentially excrete live Lassa virus in their urine. If that urine made it into the sewers, local mammals such as sewer rats could become infected and potentially establish the disease in the local area. The last thing they wanted to do was be responsible for bringing Lassa into the U.S. population.

So they decided to pour bleach, which was known to kill Lassa, into the toilets after the marines used them and let it sit long enough to decontaminate the water before flushing the toilets. However, incredibly enough, the hospital had no bleach because it was deemed a hazardous material.

Dr. Tim Burgess, a mid-grade navy infectious disease doctor with a shock of snow-white hair and a mischievous grin, got tagged to go out and get some bleach. So around midnight he drove to a grocery store in suburban Maryland and loaded up twenty-four gallons of bleach at the cash register. He says now, with a chuckle, "You get interesting looks if you show up in a military uniform at a grocery store at midnight and buy twenty-four gallons of Clorox bleach and nothing else."

The mid-twenties male cashier at the checkout counter asked him, "Eh, somethin' going on?" Tim responded, "Nah, I just needed some bleach."

Today such a purchase might prompt a terrorism alert. At the time Tim wondered how he might explain what he was doing if stopped by the cops: "It's a long story, there's this Lassa fever thing . . . ," but fortunately, he wasn't. He concluded that many unusual things happen in grocery stores at midnight or after. This was just a new wrinkle.

Meanwhile, Dr. Greg Deye in Landstuhl Germany was joined by a military preventive medicine colleague and malaria expert, Colonel Dennis Shanks, who just happened to be visiting Landstuhl for other business. Their working diagnosis for the two sick marines was Lassa fever. When they met each other in the lab and looked at the blood smears together, Dennis suddenly said, "My God, they've got malaria!"

Greg immediately called NNMC to alert his colleagues there of the possible diagnosis in the arriving marines. The NNMC docs thought it was interesting but still doubted such a large outbreak could come from malaria.

At 4:00 a.m. Sunday morning, around ten army and navy doctors, nurses, and corpsmen descended on Andrews Air Force Base in Washington DC to meet the arriving military transport plane carrying the ill marines. They had gotten word in advance of a mix of illness severity among the marines, and they were prepared with a large evacuation bus for the "walking well" and ambulances for the severely ill ones. The team was ready, wearing blue hospital gowns, N95 respirator masks, gloves, and goggles to minimize any risk of spread. One of the infectious disease fellows recalls being excited and realizing how lucky he was to get this experience, but he wondered later whether he should have been a lot more nervous.

Tim Burgess, back from his midnight store run, recalls a "surreal moment" as the back of the transport airplane opened. The flight nurses and medics on the plane, who were wearing only flight suits and no hospital protective measures, took one look at the military doctors and ran back into the plane. Had the masked and gowned docs scared them away? Not so. Moments later, they returned—armed with cameras—and snapped pictures of the doctors covered head-to-toe in their gear.

As the doctors boarded the plane, one of them recalled that the MEDEVAC team and marines stared at them as if thinking that "either they were all screwed, or we were crazy."

Even before doing complete assessments, the doctors drew blood from the sickest marines. USAMRIID Virology Division chief Dr. Tim Endy immediately drove the samples fifty miles up the road to USAMRIID to start the Lassa tests cooking.

Once in the hospital, the NNMC team decided to ferry the marines in groups up a single elevator to minimize the risk of spreading infection to others, with a plan to decontaminate the elevator afterward. They posted security guards and hospital medics on each floor to prevent other patients from using that elevator. Despite such preparation Greg Martin got a call from a nurse that a woman had just ridden up the elevator with a group of sick marines.

What?! Greg almost lost it. Would he have to quarantine a woman now for possible Lassa exposure?

The corpsman at the elevator was just trying to help the woman and hadn't wanted to keep her waiting for an elevator.

The infectious disease team set to work trying to diagnose the cause of the marines' fevers. In addition to Lassa and malaria, they considered the long list of tropical diseases that cause fever, including leptospirosis and rickettsial diseases. An experimental rapid test for malaria on ten of the marines popped up positive, providing the first indication at NNMC that some had malaria.[1]

Word of the disaster spread through the military channels and up to Colonel Bob Defraites, lead preventive medicine doctor at the army surgeon general's office. Bob, who had a long track record in field operations, sent out a prescient email: "Worried about Lassa, thinking malaria."

Later Sunday morning I received a phone call from Tim Burgess. Bad news. Some marines at NNMC were now severely ill, requiring breathing tubes, ventilators, and vasopressors to maintain their blood pressure. One marine with severe lung disease on 100 percent oxygen and a ventilator didn't look like he would make it. The team dictated an imminent death medical board and brought his mother into the room, informing her that he would probably die in a couple of hours.[2]

By this time the team had diagnosed most of the marines with malaria, but not all the puzzle pieces fit yet. The marines had been taking mefloquine. Why didn't it work? Could they have a resistant strain? Could the sickest marines be infected with both Lassa and malaria? The navy docs wanted to implement the ribavirin protocol just in case. The last thing they wanted was for the marines to survive malaria, only to die from Lassa.

I told Tim I would get the ball rolling and would meet him at USAMRIID, so he could pick up the ribavirin protocol and the drug.

It seemed simple enough . . . but not so.

I recalled approving the latest revisions to the protocol about a year earlier, and I believed that it had proceeded on its pathway through the system to approval by the FDA, which was required because ribavirin was not licensed for Lassa. However, when I asked my team for the protocol, they couldn't find the latest version.

What the hell? Where was the protocol?

After immediate scrambling and phone calls, we figured it out. The protocol had left USAMRIID, but it got lost on someone's desk at its next stop at the regulatory office at Fort Detrick. It had never made it to the FDA.

Damn! This was a major screwup.

I blamed myself for not tracking this, but there was plenty of blame to go around. After getting over our momentary panic and shouting numerous expletives, we regrouped to come up with a solution.

Fortunately, there was another way to use the drug. We picked up the phone and called the FDA person on call. After some back-and-forth, the FDA authorized emergency use of the drug (as an "emergency IND"). This didn't take too long because we already had procedures for administering the drug and we just needed the FDA's blessing. But we had egg on our faces and were embarrassed.

Fortunately we were beginning to get a better handle on what had happened. The patients started to improve on malaria treatment. One of the sickest marines at the hospital in Landstuhl appeared to have "Blackwater fever," a known complication of severe malaria. Everything pointed to malaria. The missing piece of the puzzle fell into place when Congressman John Murtha, an ex-marine himself, visited the marines on the hospital ward and the ICU. One marine confided that he and his buddies hadn't been taking their malaria pills.

Sunday night, when the Lassa tests on thirty-two marines came back negative, Sybil Tasker breathed a sigh of relief and felt as if a weight had been lifted off her shoulders. She no longer had to worry about the risk of infection spreading to others and all the logistic challenges that raised. The woman on the elevator Greg Martin had heard about would not need to be quarantined.

In the end thirty-six marines were treated on the ship, and forty-four marines were treated in the hospital for proven or suspected *Plasmodium falciparum*—the deadliest form of malaria. It was the largest outbreak of malaria in the U.S. military since the Vietnam War.

We all had dodged a bullet. No Lassa. "Only" malaria. That is like saying, "Whew, it wasn't a pipe bomb, *just* a hand grenade." Fortunately, all the marines survived—even the sickest ones, possibly because of starting malaria treatment before their arrival at the hospital.

Diseases and nonbattle injuries have caused more warrior casualties on the battlefield than bullets and bombs. Malaria usually ranks as the top or second-highest infection threat, and it has weighed heavily on U.S. military campaigns since the Revolutionary War. As a result the military has played a key role in developing all malaria drugs used in the United States—out of necessity, because of the tropical locations where military personnel are often deployed. During World War II malaria sidelined over five hundred thousand U.S. forces in Southeast Asia and the Pacific islands. General Douglas MacArthur told the army's top malaria expert at the time, "It's going to be a very long war if for every division I have facing the enemy, I have one sick in the hospital and another recovering from this dreadful disease."

As Lieutenant General William Slim, the British Corps commander during the 1943 Burma campaign, observed, "Good doctors are of no use without good discipline. More than half the battle against disease is fought, not by the doctors, but by regimental officers." By 1943–44 General Slim could measure blood levels of Atabrine, a drug to prevent malaria, so he held his commanders accountable for noncompliance among their ranks. "I only had to sack three," he said. "By then, the rest got my meaning."

Any military campaign in a tropical region of the world must contend with malaria. Dr. Dale Smith, historian at the Uniformed Services University, says, "Malaria will destroy an army, but it won't stop a war. Man's capacity to kill each other exceeds his capacity to feel ill."

There were several heroes in this story, especially the ship surgeon who recognized the parasites, which kick-started early malaria treatment for some of the marines. Also, like the desert pneumonia story, the linkages in the military infectious disease community across the globe helped.[3] Being able to pick up the phone and connect with a person you know on the other end makes a world of difference for sounding the alarm. The personal connections between army and navy physicians, USAMRIID and the hospital, and the navy hospital with its fleet all worked together to avoid what could have been a bigger disaster.

Every military disaster requires an "after action report." Dr. Charles Hoke calls the event the "4M Disaster," for marines in Monrovia with malaria who failed to take their mefloquine—a medical crisis "perfect storm." The investigation into how this chain of unfortunate events happened revealed that of the forty-four affected marines queried, few used simple measures to reduce their chances of mosquito bites: only nineteen (45 percent) used insect repellent, five (12 percent) used repellent-treated clothing, and none used bed nets. This was no surprise because no bed nets went ashore with the marines, and the shipboard stocks of permethrin for treating uniforms had been depleted. Although twenty-three (55 percent) said they complied with taking their preventive malaria pills, only a shocking four (10 percent) had levels in their blood high enough to prevent malaria. Most who admitted not taking the medicine said they just forgot.[4]

The prior deployments to areas with lower malaria risk in Iraq and Djibouti may have lulled the marines into a false sense of security and lack of awareness of the dangers awaiting in Liberia. As General Slim in the Burma campaign recognized, getting military personnel to take malaria pills only works if you watch them.

Fortunately, we occasionally learn from our failures. During the deployment to Liberia for the 2014–16 Ebola response ("United Assistance"), our experience was significantly different from the one eleven years earlier. Unit commanders required daily enforcement of taking malaria pills. The "fear factor" probably helped. Any of our soldiers who developed a fever in-country would be labeled a "possible Ebola" patient until proven otherwise. No one wanted to risk being stuck in isolation or shipped back to the United States for not taking his or her malaria pills. Sometimes other disincentives for noncompliance can improve compliance. The result was the most successful malaria prevention campaign in the history of U.S. forces. Some of the lessons from managing the marines with suspected Lassa in 2003 helped shape future design modifications at the hospital when Ebola struck in 2014–16.

So maybe we have learned something, but I can say with confidence that this isn't the last we'll hear of malaria and the military. Until we have a licensed vaccine that works, as memories of the disasters fade, more seasoned experts leave the military, and the malaria parasites become resistant to more antimalarial drugs, it is only a matter of time until the U.S. military is humbled again by malaria. Guaranteed.

5

Countermeasures

The U.S. military has been on the vanguard of defending the United States against biological weapons for over half a century, with USAM-RIID at its core. Before the anthrax attacks of 2001, USAMRIID was largely the only "game in town" in the United States developing countermeasures against biological weapons threats, from the bench top through animal models of disease and ultimately testing in humans. That has changed, as the United States has invested billions of dollars to build new laboratories and fuel research in other government laboratories, universities, and pharmaceutical companies.

Despite the popular impression that the military can get around the rules, U.S. Army programs aren't permitted to take any shortcuts when making new products and must answer to the FDA, just like everyone else.

Over decades the USAMU (U.S. Army Medical Unit) and USAM-RIID have developed an array of vaccines against numerous infectious diseases like tularemia, Q fever, Rift Valley fever virus, Staphylococcal enterotoxin B, and chikungunya.[1] Some of these were tested in the 1950s and 1960s under the classified "White Coat Program." Seventh Day Adventists who wanted to serve their country but not carry weapons volunteered as research subjects to receive experimental vaccines and undergo exposure to some of the agents. Despite the ominous sound of this testing, the program's ethical standards for informed consent of human volunteers were ahead of their time.

Hidden behind a cluster of buildings on Fort Detrick stands one of the few remaining vestiges of the United States' biological weapons program during the Cold War: a one-million-liter stainless-steel sphere, referred to as the 8 Ball, that looks like a spaceship hovering three stories above the ground. Researchers released aerosols of pathogens inside the 8 Ball to test vaccines, and the White Coat volunteers stood on a catwalk and put their faces up to external portals. As they breathed, they inhaled agents like Q fever and tularemia. Afterward doctors monitored and treated them for illness in Fort Detrick's hospital. No one died. The 8 Ball is now on the National Register of Historic Places, although some might prefer to tear it down and disavow that part of U.S. history.

Although multiple countermeasures were developed, few made it to full licensure (approval by the FDA), but the vaccines continued to demonstrate potency in regular animal testing. We continue to vaccinate laboratory workers with some of them through USAMRIID's Special Immunizations Program, which fell under my purview as chief of the Medicine Division. Multiple agencies, including elite military units and laboratory personnel elsewhere (the National Institutes of Health [NIH], the CDC, universities), have sought our vaccines to protect their laboratory workers.

Demonstrating whether a new compound works starts in the lab using tissue culture or bacterial growth inhibition. Next we move to small animals (mice, rats, guinea pigs), then maybe rabbits or monkeys to see the impact on their behavior, appetites, weight, or kidney and liver function, and whether the compound treats or protects them against infection. This can take years, but once the compound passes these major hurdles, we are not even halfway to the finish line. Now comes the much harder part: taking the compound through rigorous testing in humans to licensure by the FDA. No matter how good something looks in animals, we cannot predict how humans will react or whether the compound works. Most countermeasures fail, so licensing new drugs or vaccines can cost $1 billion and take years or decades. Large pharmaceutical companies have little enthusiasm to invest billions of dollars in vaccines or treatments against rare, high-consequence events. The low potential for profit is one reason we don't have many FDA-approved biodefense countermeasures. Developing drugs that treat chronic illnesses, like hypertension or diabetes, which must be taken long-term offer much greater profit potential.

Testing in humans runs through four phases, with increasing numbers of people receiving the new compound at each phase until we can prove the compound is safe and effective. This is a unique challenge and a significant vulnerability in biodefense and contributes to why we have few licensed vaccines and treatments against the highest bioweapon threat agents. In order to demonstrate proof of effectiveness in humans, we have to have enough people with the disease or at risk for the disease in whom we can test the product, but many of the biodefense diseases are rare. Medical ethics prevent us from doing tests such as giving people an anthrax vaccine and then infecting them purposely with deadly anthrax to see if the vaccine works.

The FDA developed the "Animal Rule" that offers a different pathway to approval, but the FDA has set a high bar. The scientific developers must produce an infection in animals that looks similar to human disease; the countermeasure has to work in animals the way we expect it to work in humans; and the countermeasure must be safe in humans. This might sound simple to achieve. It is not. Only a few compounds have been approved this way so far.

The work developing countermeasures continues, but it remains an uphill battle because our techniques are limited, the process takes years, and we can't predict what a terrorist or adversary might reach for. We have done poorly at predicting the next infectious disease challenge—even those from Mother Nature. No one envisioned a massive Ebola outbreak like the one in West Africa from 2014 to 2016, nor did we suspect Zika virus would be lurking around the corner. Everyone in public health and pandemic preparedness continues to fear that a new, deadly strain of bird flu could adapt for rapid spread between humans and cause a major pandemic like the one that killed millions in 1918.

Although we have had some recent success with promising countermeasures against Ebola, back in 2004 when Dr. Kelly Warfield accidentally stuck herself with a needle that was possibly contaminated with Ebola virus, we had very few options to choose from. We scrambled as best we could to respond.

16

The Slammer

··

DAY 0: WEDNESDAY, FEBRUARY 11, 2004

On February 11, 2004, the night of Kelly's needlestick accident, while still in the lab, she called her colleague Dianne Negley in a panic and left a message on her answering machine. Dianne has short brown hair and appears equally comfortable tanned in her running clothes or in a blue space suit. When she returned home, she heard Kelly's horrifying message: "I've had an accident and got stuck with a needle."

Diane immediately thought, *Ah shit*. She knew that Kelly had gone into the lab to work on Ebola-infected mice. She had a sinking feeling in her stomach, she recalls, "Because I knew how bad the outcome would be." She returned to the institute to help out.

Back in 2001 I had a difficult initiation my first week as the newly minted Medicine Division chief at USAMRIID. One of our virology lab technicians was working with Ebola-infected mice when he realized his laboratory space suit was partially unzipped about six inches. He reported to our clinic as a potential exposure. We considered whether he might have inhaled Ebola from the mice or their bedding. Should we put him in the Slammer? I believed the risk was too low and argued with my commander and the outgoing division chief against Slammer admission. I lost the battle. The commander decided to put the technician in the Slammer overnight.

The next morning, the Virology Division chief and a virology senior scientist confronted me in the hallway and backed me up against the wall, blaming me for the bad decision. I didn't want to throw the commander under the bus, so I took their criticism. They stirred up an internal firestorm, and the commander relented, so my team arranged for the tech's release and worked out a monitoring plan as an outpatient instead, which was what I had originally intended. He never became infected and did well in follow-up.

The episode left me a bit shaken, but I had learned some important lessons. I would never pull the trigger to put anyone in the Slammer without strong justification. I also learned to bring the relevant decision makers into the conversation early, before making a decision, and to stick to my guns if I believed I was right.

Now, three years later, Dr. Kelly Warfield had been stuck with a needle while working with Ebola-infected mice. I had the strong justification to pull the trigger. Kelly needed to go into the Slammer.

Kelly wasn't happy about getting locked up in the Slammer, "but it was the right thing to do," she said.

Despite the heart wrenching realization that she might never hug Christian, her three-year old son again, Kelly called her mom, described what had happened, and asked her to pick him up from daycare. She didn't want to risk giving him Ebola. She worried most about what would happen to Christian if she died.

When she got home, Kelly knocked on her neighbors' door. "Hi," she said. "I've just been exposed to Ebola and have to go into quarantine. Can you watch my cats for a while?" That's a great way to meet the neighbors.

A friend came over and kept her company, while Kelly stayed up all night on the phone with one of her friends and her husband, Jeremy, who was still in Texas.

After we released Kelly for the night, with a plan for her to return at 8:00 a.m. the next day, I had a heated discussion with my colleagues.

"What will Kelly do? What if she decides to skip town? How should we respond if she returns tomorrow and refuses admission to the Slammer?"

She had every right to. She was not in the military. We had no authority to retain her against her wishes.

"Would we call the police? Would the health department forcibly quarantine her?" I had no answers for any of these questions.

Before leaving USAMRIID near midnight that evening, I drafted an executive summary (EXSUM), an emergency notification for the USAMRIID commander to transmit up the army chain of command. By morning senior leaders all the way to the army surgeon general would choke on their eggs and bacon when they read it:

UNCLASSIFIED

EXECUTIVE SUMMARY

11 Feb 2004

(U) **Potential Exposure** (USAMRIID). (U) A 28-year-old female NRC fellow, with a history of rheumatoid arthritis, on multiple immunosuppressive medications, presented to the SIP clinic after sustaining a needle stick injury this afternoon while working in room AA-5 in building 1425 (BSL-4 laboratory) injecting antibody into mice that had been infected two days prior with a mouse-adapted strain of Ebola virus. After injecting antibody into four mice, she grazed the base of her left thumb with the 25-gauge needle that had been used for the prior injections. The local site bled, and she immediately decontaminated the local area with microchem [a disinfectant], saline, and betadine [an antiseptic]. The risk of exposure is categorized as probable. The risk of infection is considered low, due to the low amount of organisms thought to be present in the animals at this time with a relatively lower number of organisms that would be expected in the peritoneal tissue [the lining covering the bowel inside the abdomen], the superficial nature of the wound and the rapid wound cleansing. Special testing is being conducted on the mice to determine the levels of virus in different tissues. Based on the anticipated incubation period of the virus, there is no immediate risk to family or community contacts. The risk will be reassessed on a daily basis and the patient will be followed closely in the SIP clinic with twice daily assessments.

LTC Mark G. Kortepeter/MRMC-UIM-R/343–4994/
mark.kortepeter@amedd.army.mil

I didn't sleep well that night, haunted by images of what might happen to Kelly—feverish, disoriented, prostrate, glowing red eyes from subconjunctival hemorrhage, purpuric rash, vomiting, impending shock. In African outbreaks 100 percent of victims stuck with an Ebola-contaminated needle died. Very few infections kill a healthy person so quickly—or so efficiently.

Kelly could be the first Ebola victim ever in the United States. We really had no road map or clue how to proceed and didn't know whether anything we did could make any difference.

As I considered Kelly's near-certain death, I also wondered whether someone would blame me for letting her go home. In the government someone always takes the blame.

DAY 1: THURSDAY, FEBRUARY 12, 2004

Fortunately, we never had to deal with Kelly skipping town. One of her friends picked her up, and she arrived, surprisingly bright and fresh the next morning at 8:00 a.m., as requested.

That was the good news, but it came with a surprise. On their way in, the women had stopped at Starbucks for coffee.

Starbucks?! Shit!

I considered the timeline. We were fifteen hours from the needle-stick. *Should I worry? Could she have infected anyone?*

Probably not.

The shortest incubation period for Ebola is generally considered two days, but could we be sure? Convincing the public not to worry could be a challenge. This could easily go viral if word got out, and it would be hard to squelch a fear bonfire if the media fanned the flames. I decided to deal with that later if I had to, because we had enough to deal with at the moment.

We had prepared the Slammer overnight for Kelly's admission, setting up the room, testing the air-handling system and decon shower, and arranging round-the-clock nursing care and frequent virology lab testing. The critical care team from Walter Reed Army Medical Center arrived and filled the hallway as they unloaded boxes of equipment.

The Slammer had two patient rooms and a surgical room, as well as an anteroom. Kelly would occupy one room, another would hold equipment we would need if she got sick, and we set the third room up as a lab.

I sat down again with Kelly and the deputy commander in my

office. We told her that the plan had not changed. We would admit her to the Slammer.

We arranged for military lawyers to meet with Kelly to complete a will and advanced directives to guide life-support decisions if she was dying. Kelly took it all in stride with an upbeat and hopeful demeanor. I admired her steadiness in the face of such grave decisions.

Right after our meeting, I notified the Frederick County health officer on duty about the situation. She called me back to set up a time for a conference call with the county and state health department chiefs.

Great, I thought. *Time for a beating.*

I was suddenly a popular guy. The ringing of my office phone bore through my skull like a bad migraine. Reporters and bureaucrats in high places with titles I had never heard of managed to find my number. Like a good soldier, I referred them to our public affairs officer, Caree Vander Linden. Caree has short blond hair with little spikes, and she runs, reads, and teaches yoga in her spare time. She has a wry sense of humor, which is a job requirement after raising two teenagers and dealing with media queries for nearly a quarter century. Occasionally the reporters would call back after Caree had briefed them, begging for more details, but I felt some sinister pleasure in hanging up amid their protests, citing patient confidentiality.

Some scientists dropped by my office to argue for other home follow-up options instead of quarantining Kelly in the Slammer. I started to doubt whether I had made the right call. Should we have quarantined Kelly at home instead?

In the early afternoon, I came back to my office and noticed the message light flashing on my phone. I punched in the number to retrieve messages and heard Peter Jahrling's gravelly, Humphrey Bogart–like voice on the machine. Peter was USAMRIID's senior scientist and a top Ebola scientist. He had been at USAMRIID for over thirty years—enough to have seen multiple prior Slammer admissions. He was returning from a meeting in Boston, but he had heard about Kelly and called me from the airport.

"Mark," he greeted me. "I know some of my colleagues think Kelly should go home. I disagree. I firmly believe she belongs in the Slammer."

I respected his opinion, which made me feel a lot better about my decision.

My deputy chief and I held a conference call with the county and state health departments, and I walked them through the current situation and tried to reassure them that we had things under control. My primary goal was to ensure they would stay out of our way and not sharpshoot us when the media contacted them.

"I think we have everything covered," I said, trying not to reveal my own misgivings.

The call went smoothly—mostly. When they asked me whether Kelly had gone anywhere after leaving the institute the night before, I hesitated. *Should I tell them?* I wondered.

Then I gagged out the words, "On the way in this morning, she stopped off at Starbucks."

"Aagghhh," an anguished male voice said. I don't know who said it. It was quick but unmistakable. I braced for a string of expletives and beratement.

None came, so I ignored the sound and just drove on. "I don't think the CDC needs to be involved," I said. The last thing I needed was a bunch of armchair quarterbacks swooping in and stirring things up. They didn't agree or disagree. I don't know whether they ever called the CDC, but the CDC never called me.

I promised to keep them informed of any changes.

My colleague Colonel Jim Martin, an infectious disease doctor, agreed to serve as Kelly's primary doc while she was in the Slammer. Jim had previously jumped out of airplanes with special operations units, so he was no stranger to danger and accepted this new challenge willingly.

Kelly felt that an early care provider had avoided her like a leper, as if she already had Ebola, so now she would have a physician whom she trusted dedicated to her care. This freed me up to handle the mounting challenges outside the Slammer.

Although the Slammer was equipped with the same blue space suits as the BSL-4 laboratories, Jim and I decided that the medical team should wear standard hospital barrier protections: gowns, gloves, face shields, and an N-95 (HEPA-filtered) mask at first. Even though her risk of spreading the infection before she got sick was low, we wanted to ensure everyone followed the appropriate precautions habitually *before* Kelly got sick. The last thing we needed was for someone's careless error to force us to give Kelly a roommate. Also it was still cold and flu season, so I feared that someone could give Kelly the flu. Any fever would spell disaster, whether from influenza or some other cause, because it might force our hand to treat her for Ebola unnecessarily. We planned to upgrade to space suits if and when the time came.

We made other preparations to autoclave linens, handle garbage, and test Kelly regularly for Ebola.

Just before she entered the Slammer, Kelly emailed an invitation to her closest friends in the institute:

"Come visit (I am afraid it will be quite lonely there). . . . Please come by tonight, tomorrow, this weekend. . . . Your thoughts and prayers are MUCH appreciated."

Watching the nervous medic in the Slammer drawing her blood the first day upset Kelly. She wanted another quarantined roommate even less than we did. At her insistence her friend, Diane Negley, a medical technician with hospital experience, did all her future blood draws.

At the end of the first day of quarantine, I reflected in my office on the days' events. I thought things had gone as smoothly as I could have hoped. Starbucks seemed a distant memory.

Before I left for the day, I took a three-feet-by-four-feet piece of white art paper and drew perpendicular grid lines on it with a red magic marker. Then I taped it on my office wall and filled it in like a calendar with the days of the week for a full twenty-one days—the length of time we planned to quarantine Kelly. The day of exposure was "Day 0." Today was "Day 1."

I drew my first big red X on the February 12 square, indicating that Kelly had survived one day without a fever.

20 days to go.

DAY 2: FRIDAY, FEBRUARY 13, 2004

As each day began, I had this horrible feeling of doom—like we were prisoners marching in slow motion toward the gallows. Each day we came closer to that inevitable outcome, and I felt more scared and tense as it approached.

This morning as I entered the Medical Division wing, I noticed the Slammer door sitting wide open and medics mopping the floors inside. It took me a second to realize the disconnect.

Wait—it was closed yesterday. What the hell?

I marched down the hallway to Jim Martin's office.

"Jim, what the hell is going on? Why is the Slammer door open?" I asked. "I don't know," he said.

We quickly found the chief nurse and pulled her aside. She said that because Kelly looked fine this morning, she figured they could leave the door open.

"True, she might look fine," I said, "but that's not the point. The objective here is not to wait until she spikes a fever before sealing the door." That was like closing the barn door after the cows have left. We had no idea when Kelly would get sick, so we had to proceed as if it would happen any day.

Jim and I pulled the staff together and reeducated them about the plan. It was a sobering reminder about the challenge of communicating even among our team. We closed the door, with a plan to seal Kelly inside for nineteen more days.

That day the USAMRIID commander sent out a note to the institute to remind us to protect Kelly's privacy—a huge challenge in a close-knit institute. We had had press leaks previously.

By sheer coincidence the NIH was holding a meeting in Washington DC that week to plan a new containment laboratory to be built on Fort Detrick next to USAMRIID. I asked Colonel Scott Stanek, another division chief, to arrange a conference call with experts at the meeting. I led the call seated at the center of a large conference table surrounded by around twenty clinicians and scientists.

Although we had our own cadre of Ebola experts—Tom Geisbert, Lisa Hensley, and Peter Jahrling (who had returned from his meeting in Boston by then)—it never hurts to "phone a friend."[1]

We were desperate. We had no approved treatments. Nothing. I welcomed anything they might offer to exhaust all possible options to give Kelly the best chance of survival. The consultants on the phone included an Ebola "Who's Who." Karl Johnson and C. J. Peters were USAMRIID alumni and the "elder statesmen" in hemorrhagic fevers. Karl led the first field investigation and named Ebola for the Ebola River in northern Zaire. C.J. had helped discover the Ebola Reston virus, which was the subject of the bestseller *The Hot Zone.* Pierre Rollin from the CDC had run down numerous Ebola outbreaks in Africa. Heinz Feldmann led an Ebola research team at the Canadian containment laboratory.

Ebola outbreaks at that time occurred in remote African villages and never lasted long enough to test treatments in humans. A report from the 1995 outbreak in Kikwit, Zaire, noted that giving victims whole blood from Ebola survivors may have saved some, but the data wasn't convincing, and we had no survivor blood anyway.

During the discussion, though, Tom Geisbert mentioned that he had just completed a study treating Ebola-infected monkeys with an experimental worm protein called "rNapc2." A third of them survived, compared to the usual near-universal death rate. This was our only possible option—everything else previously tested in monkeys had failed.

Although we didn't have the magic bullet for Kelly that I would have liked, our phone conference reassured me that we hadn't missed anything. We would focus on providing the best intensive care available and just hope and pray that it might make a difference.

I was really impressed by the outpouring of support. Over the next day, I received multiple phone calls about possible treatments. The CEO of Dendreon (maker of rNapc2) called me and then shipped his product to USAMRIID.

Later that day Sina Bavari, one of our other scientists, swung by my office to discuss an "antisense" product from AVI Biopharma that had promise.[2] Ironically, Kelly had met its senior scientist at a seminar the day of her accident. The compounds were small pieces of DNA with complementary genetic sequences that attach, like Lego blocks, to the virus genes and shut down replication. The company tailor-made some against Ebola and shipped them to us.

At the end of the day and a few steps closer to the gallows, I made my second red *X* on my calendar for February 13.

Nineteen days to go.

That evening during my drive home, Peter Jahrling called me. "Mark. Tony Fauci wants to talk to you." "Tony Fauci? Are you kidding me?"

Dr. Anthony Fauci, director of the National Institute of Allergy and Infectious Diseases (NIAID) at the NIH and one of the most powerful and well-regarded scientists in the field of infectious diseases wanted to speak with *me*? The idea of talking to Tony prompted a visceral fear of being called to the principal's office. *What was I going to tell him? Would he second-guess me?*

Nevertheless, after I got home, I sat down at my desk, drafted a couple of preparatory notes, and called him at home. To my surprise he put me at ease immediately—like talking to another physician on hospital rounds. In his characteristic Brooklyn accent, he offered assistance with possible use of an Ebola DNA vaccine that the NIAID was testing. He referred me to the head of its clinical trials unit, who gave me some additional information about the vaccine, which was undergoing early safety (phase 1) testing in humans, but it had a long way to go before testing whether it worked in humans.

I appreciated the offer, but I was reluctant to use it because it had failed to protect monkeys from Ebola. Kelly's situation set a much higher bar—trying to prevent illness *after* she had already been infected. Kelly had rheumatoid arthritis, and I feared the vaccine might rev up her immune system and worsen her disease or cause other unexpected side effects. I didn't want to give her something that we might later regret, unless it showed great promise. I decided, though, to let Jim Martin and Kelly make the final decision as doctor and patient.

Even if we wanted to, we couldn't just pick something and give it. We had to establish an "emergency IND" with the FDA and convince the agency that any unlicensed products promised to help the patient with a low risk of harm and that it really was an emergency. Fortunately, that was not too difficult. We drafted a couple of short experimental protocols and consent forms, and we conferred with the FDA officer on call. Within hours, we had the approvals for using any of the products, if needed.

While I dealt with administrative and regulatory hassles on the outside, Kelly sweated it out inside the Slammer. To compound her fear of Ebola and being cut off from the world, Kelly had personal issues to deal with. Her husband, Jeremy, flew in hastily from Texas, where he had been doing army training for several weeks. The army had transferred him the prior year to Georgia. He had received promises of returning eventually to Walter Reed Army Medical Center in Washington DC, but things were not going as planned. I was really impressed when our commanding general met with Kelly and Jeremy in the Slammer fully garbed in protective gear. He offered a sympathetic ear and promised to contact someone regarding Jeremy's assignment.

It really helped having a knowledgeable patient who could make informed decisions about her treatment. On the day of her admission, Kelly plunked down a stack of Ebola articles on Jim Martin's desk for him to read as her physician. Once we had collected information on the three possible products, Jim and Kelly conferred. The vaccine was taken off the table as unlikely to provide benefit. We decided to wait on giving either of the other products until Kelly showed signs of infection, like a fever or abnormal labs. This way we stood by one of medicine's oldest promises to patients: "primum no nocere" (first do no harm).

Day 3: Saturday, February 14, 2004, and Beyond

The night of Kelly's accident, Diane Negley had returned to the institute to help collect the mice that Kelly had worked on for urgent harvesting and testing. We needed to know whether Kelly's mice had Ebola virus growing in them at the time of her needlestick.

"There were a lot of unknowns," Diane says. "The probability [of infection] was lower end, but you still didn't know until you tested the animals." Using initial PCR testing, only one of the ten mice Kelly had worked with tested positive at low levels—and none of the four mice Kelly had injected had detectable virus. So far so good.

However, in a second round of more sensitive tests, four of the mice had detectable virus. We had a legitimate cause for concern. It was no longer theoretical.

We took some grief when others were shocked, *shocked* that Kelly had been working in BSL-4 while on medications for her rheumatoid arthritis, but that eventually blew over. As word spread up the chain, though, the commander and I were summoned to the Pentagon to meet with the deputy assistant secretary of defense (DASD) for safety and occupational health. As we passed by a sea of offices in the Pentagon searching for the right one, I felt increasingly annoyed at wasting several hours just to hold some bureaucrat's hand when I had a patient to worry about.

We finally shuffled into a small, austere room with about ten people seated around a small conference table. I couldn't fathom why any of them had any business being there.

I barely had a chance to pull up the chair of "honor" next to the overweight secretary with the Fred Flintstone face when he said, "Why did you let her go home?"

I didn't feel like taking any crap and went into offensive mode, firing back, point by point, the reasons for our decision. I emphasized that we took appropriate steps to minimize risk to the public, and our actions had to stand up to scrutiny from the *scientific and the medical* communities, not to rumor and innuendo. I conveniently left out the visit to Starbucks. I was pleased that my commander chimed in several times and defended me. The DASD seemed satisfied, and the meeting didn't last long.

At this point, three days into the incubation period, we had the possible treatments in the freezer. Now began an excruciating period of waiting, crossing our fingers, hoping, and praying.

My wife's birthday came and went without any celebration. Sadly, she was used to having my patients come first. Next year would be different I promised.

With each successive square I crossed out on my calendar, I felt better, but the time went by very slowly.

Every day brought new challenges.

The Walter Reed Army Medical Center, fearful of contagion, refused to accept routine labs, despite a long-standing agreement to do so, so we had to spin up a lab system and blood bank quickly inside the Slammer.

How were we to feed Kelly? We worked out a system where Kelly ordered take-out from local restaurants, then one of her friends would pick it up, don protective equipment, and bring the food in to Kelly. She became particularly fond of sushi.

Also we had a plan to clean bed linens, but no plan for her personal laundry. Kelly improvised by washing her clothes in the sink and drying them in the tub. Unfortunately, the stiffened clothes irritated her skin.

Kelly's rheumatologists recommended that we stop all her rheumatology medications, but doing so caused painful flare-ups in her hands that Jim treated with ibuprofen and acetaminophen with codeine for additional pain control. Ironically, since Ebola triggers a massive, detrimental immune response (known as a "cytokine storm"), we wondered whether Kelly's usual medications that suppressed her immune system might help by dampening the body's hyper-response to Ebola. However, we decided not to risk testing that hypothesis.

Kelly had numerous visitors. Although it helped her peace of mind, I was concerned that when she became ill, or if we had a mishap, we might have to lock up more people. We tracked the date and time anyone entered the unit, but on February 15 (Day 4), we cracked down. Kelly was approaching the period of highest risk for spiking a fever from Ebola, so we asked her to choose only six possible visitors, and we would exclude everyone else. She was not happy, but she understood that if we had to quarantine both of her parents, Christian would have no caregiver. She made the heart-wrenching decision to exclude her father.

As I crossed out each daily calendar box, Kelly dealt with her own private hell. She spent the first week on edge, fearful of getting sick, and haunted by images of dying monkeys she had infected. She envisioned having the same fate and didn't want such a painful, terrible death.

"Just give me morphine, keep me comfortable," she pleaded with her husband.

Despite her fears she didn't want her death to be a waste. She wanted the medical team to take a lot of specimens and conduct an autopsy. Maybe knowledge gained from her death could make a difference for someone else.

Kelly also felt as if she were living inside a fishbowl, with multiple people monitoring her every move. She requested Ambien regularly to sleep.

None of Kelly's early tests showed activation of her immune system, so around the end of the first week, she began to feel hopeful things would be okay. On February 17 (Day 6), Kelly sent a note to her colleagues: "I was PCR negative yesterday and all my other tests look great. . . . I'm feeling great and in good spirits."

I was not so optimistic. The usual incubation period is about eight to twelve days. I wasn't ready to pop the champagne cork yet.

Kelly began her next phase: feeling stir crazy. She wanted just to scream, "Let me out of here!"

On February 18 (Day 7) she emailed the deputy commander: "I am using the cards to decorate my room. It's pretty boring looking at concrete walls all day. . . . However, I am doing great!"

On the same day she emailed her friend Julie Boyer: "We'll be dancing tonight, if the tests come back clean today." Julie responded, "Do you remember how badly we dance?"

Nevertheless, after taking a shower the next day, she noticed a rash on her arm. Worried, because rash is an early sign of infection, she called her doctor, Jim Martin, in the middle of the night. Could it be Ebola? He was less concerned because she didn't have any other new symptoms and nothing else had changed. He examined her the next morning. The rash resolved on its own over the next couple of days.

Another night late in the evening, when no one was around, Kelly told the nurses to contact facilities because she was feeling warm and needed the room temperature changed. When the facilities crew member got the call, he rushed down to the Slammer, afraid that something was wrong, that Kelly was sick or had a fever. It turns out, Dianne Negley explained, "She just wanted to talk to somebody."

Kelly had hoped to remain anonymous, but on February 19 someone in the institute leaked the news to the press. Kelly was particularly incensed that the detailed description in the news might allow someone to identify her. We had already drafted a press release just in case, so we launched it immediately. The commander followed up with a second email to the institute: "This is a reminder that all press inquiries should be referred to Ms. Caree Vander Linden or Mr. Chuck Dasey. Violation of our policy in this regard could make you liable for punishment or dismissal. . . . This Command will have a zero tolerance for release of private and sensitive information."

On that same day, Kelly wrote to some friends: "Information about the Ebola exposure was leaked to the press. Trying to stay positive. I'm almost out of the darkest part of the woods!" and "the last 7 days weren't that bad because it's been the waiting game each day. . . . The next 14 are going to be hard."

The exposure made the local and national headlines, but our army public affairs officers wouldn't let me talk to the press. This annoyed me because it left a vacuum of information, so the news channels went elsewhere for their information. The CDC supported us. It never hurts to have a vote of confidence from the "big boys." My decision to talk with the county and state health departments was validated. Without that we probably would have taken more heat for sending Kelly home that first night. ABC News got the story wrong, though, saying the patient was feeling ill the day after the accident. Our public affairs officers sent a corrective note, but I'm not sure whether the network ever issued a correction.

Kelly was determined to use her time in isolation to work, but it wasn't easy. On February 19 (Day 8), she emailed a friend: "I think that work is the only way I'm going to get through the next 2 weeks. The last week has been tough, just waiting . . . hard to concentrate."

The highlight of her days became her morning blood draws, when she and Diane Negley would share coffee and breakfast, afternoon visits with PCR results from Lisa Hensley or Elizabeth Fritz, and the evenings, when Diane returned with another friend, Dana Swenson, for dinner.

For Diane and her other friends, the possibility that Kelly might die was on their minds early on because, as she noted, "We all knew one PFU [plaque forming unit] could kill her."[3]

Considering the circumstances Diane thought Kelly was dealing with the situation very well. Even though she knew Kelly was feeling bad, Diane said, "You didn't hear her complain. You could just see in her face and her movements how she was hurting." Diane spent a lot of time "just being her friend" and letting her "talk about whatever she wanted to talk about."

As each day passed, watching the rooms in the Slammer fill up with new equipment intended for her care unnerved Kelly: a ventilator; dialysis, ultrasound, and X-ray machines; an on-site laboratory, and a blood bank. She had to climb around equipment just to look out the window.

Using PCR we hoped to identify whether Kelly had virus growing in her blood before she felt any symptoms to give us a head start on treating her. PCR can detect extremely low levels of virus, but this advantage brings a downside risk of a *false positive*, meaning that the test is positive, but the patient is not infected. As a self-check we ran the tests in two different labs, one in virology and one in diagnostics.

We drew Kelly's blood every morning, and much to the chagrin of the physicians, Kelly's friends in the lab bypassed the usual information chain and phoned her or walked down to the Slammer in the afternoon to tell her the lab results, speaking loudly at the window of the Slammer door.

One afternoon in the first ten days, we had a bombshell. Kelly received a call from Lisa Hensley. The test for Ebola in one lab was *positive!* "Don't freak out," Lisa said. The test in the other lab was negative. "We're re-running the tests."

This really tightened our sphincters. Was Kelly infected? Split lab results could indicate a low level of virus . . . or contamination in the lab.

Fortunately, on the repeat assessments, both tests were negative.

We all breathed a sigh of relief . . . until we were jolted temporarily by another false positive later.

On February 21 (Day 10) Kelly received an email from the institute commander suspending her laboratory access . . . indefinitely, "pending a review of [her] medical condition."

She was crushed and angry. Diane said she was "a little furious."

The delivery of the commander's message by email, rather than on the phone or in person, particularly angered her.

Kelly fired off a note to Nancy Jaax, former Pathology Division chief and a pioneer for women working in BSL-4. "Nan—They've pulled my suite access. . . . Gee, he could have waited until a better time, you think? . . . Right now I am freaking out. He just decimated my life in one email."

So compounded with the fear of death and feeling isolated, Kelly now faced the end of her professional research career. Her future hung in limbo. Fortunately, she had some advocates in the institute. She received a reassuring note from the deputy commander that he would ensure the situation was handled fairly and impartially. In a subsequent note to Nancy Jaax, Kelly wrote, "My knight in shining armor [the deputy commander] has appeared. . . . At least someone is looking out for me."

By the time I crossed out Day 14 (February 25) in red marker on my makeshift calendar, I felt the veil of gloom lifting. Kelly felt this as well. Two days later, she sent a note out to the institute inviting everyone to "come celebrate freedom."

Jim Martin's note in her medical chart on March 1 (Day 19) notes, "Exam unchanged (except for painted nails)." Clearly, Kelly was getting ready for a "jail break."

As the mood began to lighten inside the Slammer, Diane brought in some beer one night. As the beer went through the security scanner, the guard said, "Heineken?" "No, Fosters," Diane said. "Tell Kelly we said hi," he told her.

Another night, near the end, the women shared some champagne.

I am glad I didn't know about it, otherwise I might have had to intervene and spoil the celebration. After all it was a government facility and alcohol was not permitted.

DAY 21: WEDNESDAY, MARCH 3, 2004

After twenty-one days in quarantine, we freed Kelly. We all felt as if we had received a stay of execution. The institute held a party that afternoon, complete with snacks and balloons. She and nurse friend Denise Clizbe put together a mock newsletter with the headline: "Prisoner Released from the Slammer!" featuring a photo of a smiling Kelly looking out through the Slammer door's window. The day after discharge, she received a medical bill from the army for $267.00. It was later rescinded.

To this day she retains copies of all the emails and cards from well-wishers that she received while in containment.

There were no hugs in front of CNN cameras, however. Kelly could have gone on the talk-show tour and made a lot of money, but she preferred to stay out of the news, fearing potential negative impact on her career or being viewed as exploiting the situation.

Despite her release her ordeal would continue for several more months. I assigned one of my physicians to do a comprehensive medical evaluation, so we could give the commander adequate justification to let her back into the lab. I feel proud that we did it, and the commander eventually approved her return. Barring her from the lab would have been tragic. Kelly's scientific career continues to thrive in her new role leading research in a private company—still on Ebola. Her husband, Jeremy, was reassigned back to Walter Reed the next year and eventually became chief of Oncology. She has a large family with three stepchildren and two new children, ages two and four. Christian, the three-year-old boy during this ordeal, is now eighteen. It is unlikely that he remembers this scary time.

When I asked her recently, Kelly said that I needn't have worried about her skipping town that first night before her slammer admission. She never considered it. "Where would I have gone, anyway?" Good question. If she had been infected with Ebola, she would have surfaced somewhere.

After Kelly's discharge I saw it as a perfect opportunity to turn a negative story into a positive one for USAMRIID. The commander agreed to let us invite in the media. We gave several reporters a good "dog and pony" show describing the institute's capabilities and research activities and answered all their questions, followed by a tour of the Slammer. They wrote positive stories.

A couple of years later, a group of us from the organizations that had built specialized sites for care of patients with Ebola and other highly hazardous infectious diseases, including USAMRIID, Emory University, and the University of Nebraska, met to draft guidelines on containment care for patients ("biocontainment").[4] Kelly provided a valuable perspective to that discussion. Several new BSL-4 laboratories were popping up in the post-9/11 world, so I wanted to ensure that others could learn from our experience. We published an article, with Kelly as one of the coauthors, that included a list of all historic Slammer admissions.[5] I shared this several years later with German colleagues who faced a similar tragedy in their Hamburg lab.

Only two and a half months after Kelly exited the Slammer, we had a very sobering reminder of the gravity of our situation. On May 24, 2004, Russia announced that Antonina Presnyakova, chief lab technician of the Division of Highly Dangerous Pathogens of the Institute of Molecular Biology at the State Research Center of Virology and Biotechnology ("Vector") in Novosibirsk, had a presumed needlestick injury while working in the lab on Ebola.

She became infected and died.

On the Hot Side

··

In the spring of 2004, I started getting calls from colleagues asking me when I would leave USAMRIID, because they wanted my job. USAMRIID helped me find my passion for infectious diseases and my niche in biodefense. I didn't want to return to general public health work. So a couple of months after Kelly's Ebola scare and after five and a half years at USAMRIID, I left for three years of specialized infectious disease training at the army's lead hospital, Walter Reed Army Medical Center, in Washington DC. When I completed my fellowship in 2007, it was natural for me to return "home" to USAMRIID, but I sought a different experience this time. I had worked as a lab technician for a year before medical school, so I felt comfortable in the lab as well as in the hospital. Undeterred by Kelly's Slammer experience, I wanted my own opportunity to work on the "hot side." I asked to be assigned to the Virology Division.

Most prior Ebola animal studies tested new vaccines and treatments or assessed Ebola's destruction of major body organs. In the absence of a magic bullet, which seemed years away, we had no idea of the best way to take care of Ebola patients. Some believed that treating Ebola victims was futile if most are destined to die anyway. In the first outbreak of Marburg in 1967, 23 percent of patients in Germany and Yugoslavia died, whereas fatality rates in later outbreaks in the Democratic Republic of Congo and Angola had reached 83–90 percent. This gave some indication that intensive care for Ebola or Marburg-infected patients could be beneficial, but we didn't know what aspect might make a difference. As a physician, I brought a unique perspective to help bridge the divide between what we could study in monkeys and humans. I jumped at the chance to get in on the ground level of Ebola research. So, assisted by an expert team of Ebola scientists and technicians, I picked up a monkey Ebola research project from a colleague. The project pushed into unexplored territory: determining what happened during the disease on a minute-by-minute basis and whether something as simple as intravenous fluids could save the monkeys.[1] I was thrilled to be back in science and working on something that might help patients.

It sounds simple, but it was far from it. You can't just take a blood pressure on an Ebola-infected monkey like you might on a human. Monkeys don't let you get close. To get around this challenge, we implanted sensors inside the animals, so we could measure their heart and lung function. Antennae placed inside the cages picked up signals from the sensors, which we recorded at a base station outside the lab. Next, we inserted intravenous catheters, so we could give IV fluids and draw blood without anesthetizing the animals. In severely ill animals, sedating drugs could tip the balance toward death prematurely and alter the parameters we measured.

First we measured baseline vital signs on each monkey (heart rate, blood pressure, temperature, breathing rate); then we infected the monkeys with Ebola and watched whether giving some monkeys extra boluses of IV fluid made a difference in their survival.

Every morning I stopped by the lab and peered through a narrow window to eyeball how my first three monkeys were doing. Early on they looked at me with curious, bright eyes. By day six fever had struck, and they slowed down, stopped eating, and became less aggressive.

Today was the eighth day after infection. From the window I had trouble seeing the monkeys because they were sick and hunkering down in the rear of their cages. Next, I stopped by our monitoring station behind the lab. Like an intensive-care doctor monitoring his patients' vital signs in the ICU, I scanned across four TV monitors and the squiggly lines of red and blue moving across the screens. I scrolled through the real-time values of the vital signs for all three animals, as well as their overnight readings, looking for trends. The animals' blood pressure tracings were heading on a downward arc at the same time that their heart rates rocketed skyward in tandem with their breathing rates. It was a thrill just to see this pattern emerging that no one had documented before or measured in real time in Ebola-infected monkeys or humans. I saved the data on a computer disk for further analysis.

As I would do with my patients in the hospital, once armed with the basic vital signs on my monkeys, I needed to see them up close to make a "bedside" assessment.

Time to enter the lab.

Like a pilot performing a preflight test, I follow a standardized process before each entry into the maximum containment (BSL-4) lab. The twenty-minute pre-entry ritual starts in the locker room, where I strip down to bare skin, remove my wedding ring and watch, and pull on a pair of white scrubs and socks.

I tiptoe through the shower, in case the floor is wet from prior use. Then I pass through a door into the "gray" or "warm" side, a weigh station the size of a small coffee kiosk between the "cold" side locker room and the "hot" lab.[2] Here is my last chance for a bathroom break before entering containment.

Wrapping my wrists and ankles with autoclave tape, I seal the gap between my socks and pant legs, as well as between my purple nitrile gloves and sleeves.[3] Before putting it on, I inspect my blue space suit closely for tears or holes, paying close attention to the weak spots around the windshield-like face mask, the moving joint areas, and especially the gloves and air tubes. I insert earplugs as my last step before stepping inside the suit, like a fireman putting on heavy fireproof clothing. Next I slide one hand in, then duck inside while wriggling in the other arm. With my right hand, I pull the thick rubber zipper closed from my left shoulder to my right hip, tracing the seal with my left hand to ensure closure. Any gap in the zipper could allow entry of lab air into the suit and risk exposure to a pathogen.

I grab the end of a tightly coiled, yellow plastic hose dangling from the ceiling and insert it with a "snap" into a valve on my suit, trying not to catch my gloves between the two ends. A "glove break" now would force me to start all over.

As the cool rush of air hisses into the suit, like an inflating tire, it brings with it a plastic scent of polyvinyl chloride. The suit around me inflates slowly, like a beach ball, until I feel the sides push up against my arms.

With the suit partially inflated, I feel secure that there are no major leaks and am ready to leave the gray side. The large stainless-steel shower door looms ahead of me, like the watertight barrier between compartments on a submarine. I feel nervous anticipation in the pit of my stomach. Once beyond that barrier, there is no easy escape.

I uncouple my air hose, and the hissing stops abruptly. I punch in a security code next to the shower, and a button with a red light turns green. All clear to enter. The electron magnet releases the door with a "clunk" sound. I wait another five seconds, watching rubber inflatable gaskets around the door deflate before opening. The solid steel door takes considerable effort to pull open and similar effort to slow its opening momentum.[4]

I step into the decontamination shower, about the size of a freight elevator. A steamy residue hangs in the air, like a morning fog, from a prior user. The closing door makes another loud clunk as the electron magnet engages behind me. I don't turn on the shower yet. On the way into the lab, the shower only serves as a conduit to the hot side. After I push the exit button on the opposite side, another red button turns green, and a magnetic lock releases a second door. I step through and before closing it, trigger the shower to start a decon cycle, to sterilize the air in the shower for the next lab worker. The door clicks shut, and the shower whooshes on.

The shower goes through its seven-minute cycle before anyone can enter or exit.

No turning back now.

Welcome to the hot side.

I feel safe in this oasis of silence, free from the daily hassles of meetings, phones, and email. Just science.

After donning heavy green rubber boots to protect my feet, I waddle down the central corridor of the suite, like a pregnant woman in her third trimester, passing several laboratory rooms on either side and walls and ceilings covered with a maze of pipes, wires, and tubes. Yellow coiled air hoses hang from the ceiling at programmed intervals. A blue strobe light, like the K-Mart "blue light special," hangs in the center of the ceiling next to a yellow strobe light, a blue egg-shaped video camera, and sprinkler valves. The hissing airflow at eighty decibels, along with the earplugs, makes verbal communication inside the lab nearly impossible, so each light has its own special function: Blue signals to watch for an urgent message on an electronic marquee. Yellow means get out of the lab immediately because the air may run out.

We have adopted ways to communicate in containment. Sometimes we cheat and pinch the air hose to stop the airflow momentarily. The safety folks don't like this because it can damage the air hoses, but it works in a "pinch." We can also write on a dry erase board to communicate through a window with someone in the outside hallway. Some places use wireless headsets. When all else fails, we shout or use hand signals.

As I unhook between air hoses to move down the corridor or around the lab, the suit holds a couple of minutes of air inside, so I can move freely until the visor fogs up, signaling it's time to hook up again for fresh air.

Hearing is not the only sense diminished in the name of protection. Through two layers of gloves, I lose my fine touch as if I were wearing dishwashing gloves. Because the hands are the most vulnerable part of the suit, I move them with deliberate slowness. My visual field is similarly impaired, and I can't see through the visor beyond ninety degrees to the right or left without turning my body, like someone with a stiff neck. The worst is not being able to scratch an itch. Some petite women can pull their arms back inside the suit and scratch, but I am not so agile.

At the end of the corridor, I turn right into an animal room as large as a good-sized bedroom. Four stainless steel monkey cages, two to a row, stacked on top of each other, sit against the wall to my left and in front of me. I can barely hear, but the monkeys against the wall in front of me generally don't make much noise.

Rhesus macaques are midsize monkeys, bigger than a beagle and smaller than a Labrador retriever. Covered with dusty brown or auburn fur, they have hairless pink faces with closely set eyes and elongated noses, similar to characters in *Planet of the Apes*. Rhesus macaques are common faces in scientific labs, because they are easy to keep in captivity and they adapt well to human company. They are anatomically and physiologically similar to humans, which is why we use them extensively in experiments related to human health.

Even ill monkeys can be vicious and grab or scratch me from the cage without warning. So I observe them from a safe distance to document today's examination—their activity levels, skin rashes, eye redness, how much fruit or biscuits they have eaten, or whether there is visible urine in the large collection pan under the cages.

Trained to avoid direct eye contact (a behavior that piques dominant behavior in the wild), I can nonetheless see, through averted eyes, their pink gums pulling back exposing white fangs, but with a more tentative threat than yesterday. My monkeys, eight days into infection, show signs of severe illness. They have a blank stare, as they crouch in the back corners of their cages, holding their abdomens. One has scattered, tiny red dots (petechiae) on its face and inner thighs. Their groins, swollen from fluid, look like overfilled water balloons.

Today I notice something different, though. Two of the monkeys don't look good, but the third, which had appeared to be on a downward spiral twenty-four hours ago, appears to have perked up. This is extremely rare. Once on a downward glide, most monkeys eventually succumb to infection. When it is clear they have reached the point of no recovery, our ethical guidelines call for euthanasia.

Once done making my notes, I follow the standard sequence out of the lab—a full decon shower, removal of the space suit, and a personal soap-and-water shower. After I have dressed, I return to the base station to review the latest parameters on the animals. The values confirm what I saw. The squiggly red and blue lines for one animal show a declining heart rate and stabilizing blood pressure. Could this animal be recovering? I was so excited at what this animal's data could show us that I emailed my team as soon as I could: *If I were in the hospital and this monkey were my patient, I would be jumping for joy right now!*

Over approximately one year, we assessed the response of nine monkeys infected with Ebola virus. We had a very unusual result: three survivors. Only one of the survivors had received intravenous fluid treatment. Two had received no intervention, so the fluids didn't improve the chances of survival, but the extraordinary finding was that all the animals that received extra fluids preserved their kidney function, even if they still died. Wow! Such a basic concept but never tested with Ebola. If we could preserve one major organ using only IV fluids, perhaps adding other interventions might preserve more organs or improve survival rates. We also documented for the first time the differences in vital sign changes during illness between monkey Ebola survivors and nonsurvivors.[5] Our data was pure—not influenced by any medicines. Perhaps that knowledge could someday lead to improved care for infected humans.

I have a natural paranoia about infectious diseases—probably not a bad thing when working in a containment lab. It's important to have a healthy respect for the power of deadly microbes, but sometimes your mind can play tricks on you when you step back and consider how close you come to some nasty things. The space suit may seem like overkill, until you remind yourself that the smallest drop of secretions from an infected monkey contains millions of virus particles, and it only takes a few to kill you.

One time, while holding a sedated monkey severely ill from Ebola, the monkey reached up and tapped my gloved hand. I didn't think anything of it until later that day outside the lab, when I noticed a scratch on my finger.

Was it there before?

Was that the finger the animal touched?

Was that even the same hand?

Could that little tap have scratched me?

I felt reasonably sure that the monkey didn't cause it, but I had just enough doubt to feed my paranoia. That experience reminded me to remain extra vigilant when assessing my gloves to ensure they had no holes or cuts.

Another time, while on a family trip, I awoke in the hotel in the middle of the night frightened by a dream that I had had a lab accident with Ebola. My three-year-old son was asleep in the next bed. In my semiconscious fog, I noticed a line of blood across his face coming from his ear. "Oh my God," I thought. "He's got Ebola!" I jumped out of bed and was about to shake him awake when I realized that he had a bloody nose, probably from the dry air in the hotel. The line of blood had dripped from his nose down across his cheek to his ear. I felt foolish and crawled back into bed, but I had difficulty getting back to sleep.

Later that year I presented our research findings at an international meeting of Ebola experts in Japan. At the end of my presentation, Ebola legend Karl Johnson—the man who named the virus—spoke up from the audience with the ultimate compliment: "Mark," he said, "the data you presented is probably the most detailed that we will likely ever have [on Ebola]."

I was caught off guard and managed only to stammer, "Thank you, Karl," but that is when I realized the true significance of our research.

But this was just the beginning. Like every good experiment, our study also raised important new questions: Is there an optimal amount of fluids we should give? Should we give the fluids all at once or gradually? Could we combine fluids with other countermeasures to preserve more major organs or decrease the death rate? Why does the blood pressure fall?

Answers to those questions would have to wait for another day, because I received a call from our commanding general that would have an important impact on the next phase of my career. The army had bigger plans in store for me than doing Ebola research.

18

Descent into Hell

It was the spring of 2008. I sat in lotus position with the warm sun at my back in a grassy field next to the woods—a refreshing alternative to the office or a space suit. The night before I had slept out under the stars with only a sheet of plastic for shelter, a sleeping bag, and a liter of water. This morning I was directed to meditate on my place in the world for four hours.

My fifteen-year-old-son, Luke, sat next to me and appeared lost in thought. We were at Little Bennett State Park in Maryland, undergoing the initiation rites for the Order of the Arrow, an elected group in Boy Scouts that performs community service.

I was deep in my head, wrestling with a decision that would dramatically change my career path. Our commanding general had tapped me to serve as the next deputy commander of USAMRIID—the second-highest position at the institute, running the daily operations, like a chief operating officer. It's a tough job. The institute had grown to eight hundred employees, with a $125 million budget, and held a stockpile of vaccines, antidotes, and trillions of virulent microbes that literally have a life of their own.

I wasn't sure I wanted the job, so I appreciated the silent time to navigate my professional crossroads while ignoring the dew seeping into my pants.

At this point I had made it to my "terminal" rank as a full "bird" army colonel, meaning I wore an eagle symbol on my shoulders. I had no designs on bucking for the next promotion to general.

Previously, when the army had offered me a new assignment, I saluted and made the best of it. As a colonel I had flexibility to choose my assignments, without fear of repercussions. But it's hard to turn down a general, especially one with whom I had served with previously. In some ways the job offered everything I had strived for since my arrival at USAMRIID, and it would fulfill a core ambition to do something important. On the other hand, it would pull me away from my blossoming Ebola research and back into the endless quandaries of leadership.

My three boys would invariably get short-changed by the job. My oldest son, Luke, would be driving in a year, and I enjoyed listening to his growing mastery of the piano and watching his cross-country races. Sean, ten, and Daniel, five, both loved swimming and played the violin. My wife, Cindy, a pharmacist, was a team leader at the FDA. She had already borne her share of solo parenting during my overseas deployments and multiple other travels.

I was reluctant to pass up the opportunity, though, to help run the nation's lead biodefense research institute. By the time the sun rose on the second morning at Little Bennett, I made my final decision. I would take the job.

Little did I know that this decision would carry me to the gates of hell. The change of command took place on June 24, 2008. The purgatory that began just sixteen days later, ironically, on a day of celebration at USAMRIID, would prove just as "hot" and challenging as any of the work inside the labs.

U.S. military forces received a plague vaccine during the Vietnam war because Vietnam is one of the world's hot spots for one Chessman: Bishop Plague. The vaccine prevented the form of plague spread by fleas, bubonic plague, which kills about two-thirds of its victims. The much deadlier (nearly 100 percent fatal) pneumonic plague infects victims through the air straight into their lungs, which is the route of choice for a bioweapon. Like a wildfire once the infection begins, it propagates from one victim to another without fleas.

The old vaccine used in Vietnam had a couple of problems. It was made by growing a soup of plague, like growing yeast to make beer, and then killing the organism with formalin. This mixture was then injected into the arm muscle. I've had two doses of the vaccine, so

I can personally attest that it hurt like hell, in addition to other side effects, like headache and malaise.

But the main reason we needed a new vaccine was because the old one would fail to protect our military forces from an airborne bioweapon attack. Our job was to come up with a new vaccine to ensure that the Black Death never got inside a soldier, airman, or marine through their lungs.

USAMRIID's new vaccine was called F1-V, named after different proteins (antigens) that the plague bacteria make to get around our body's natural defenses. It secretes a sticky substance that contains the F1 antigen that surrounds and protects the organism from our body's white blood cell "Pac men." V is another antigen that pulls toxic substances produced by plague inside the cell and suppresses our body's immune response. The vaccine gives us a head start in the battle to produce antibodies against those antigens, which bind to and neutralize the organism's deadly cascade.

Our vaccine had overcome a critical hurdle and protected monkeys against pneumonic plague. So on July 10, 2008, we had a celebration at the institute because things looked promising to advance the vaccine through the complex pathway toward licensure. I was proud of our scientists and happy to be part of the celebration. After two weeks on the job, I also felt gratified that I had developed the right skillsets of leadership, clinical knowledge, and scientific credibility over my career to be effective as the deputy commander.

We invited the scientists who had developed the vaccine to the celebration, along with company representatives who would take the vaccine to the next, more difficult level—to cross what is called "the valley of death" from animal testing through human testing, where most new vaccines reach a dead end.

The USAMRIID commander opened the ceremony, followed by several speakers who discussed the science and the planned future studies.

Early in the ceremony, I noticed my colleague Lieutenant Colonel Bret Purcell walk down the aisle to my right and tap Bruce Ivins on the shoulder. With a medium build and short, straight brown hair, Bret was an avid historian and traveler and an anthrax and plague physician/scientist in the Bacteriology Division. Bruce was one of our senior bacteriology scientists and an expert on anthrax and anthrax vaccines. He had short, light brown hair, a quirky smile, and a lopsided gait. Bret and Bruce were friends. Bret leaned over and whispered something to Bruce, who stood up, and they shuffled off together. I did not think much of it at that moment, but Pat Worsham, who by then had been promoted to chief of the Bacteriology Division, noted that Bret's normal steady facial expression "looked anguished." She suspected something was up.

A short time later, while the celebration continued, the commander's secretary came up and handed me a note. She appeared a bit flustered, and she whispered that the commander had been called to an urgent meeting across the base. Before leaving he had asked if I could close the celebration and hand out a few USAMRIID coins to the visiting speakers.

"No problem," I said. "I'll be happy to close the meeting."

The secretary also said that after the celebration, I should drop by Lieutenant Colonel Demmin's office. Lieutenant Colonel Demmin was our chief of safety, security, plans and operations, who managed the paperwork and informed the chain of command about lab mishaps. The secretary didn't know the reason, but she said, "It might have something to do with an exposure," and that Pat Worsham should accompany me. I suspected she meant a lab exposure. I had dealt with Ebola, anthrax, and plague exposures as the Medical Division chief, so there was little that could faze me. I suspected that if it had been a critical exposure, I would have been informed immediately, and I was confident my personnel in Medical Division could handle something routine.

Refocusing my thoughts on the celebration, I immediately jotted a couple of notes to myself on what to say, including who I needed to give coins to. "Coining" is a long military tradition that allows a commander to thank visitors who have done something for their unit by giving them a coin with the unit's symbol on it. Military people display these coins proudly in their offices or on their desks. I have a collection of about thirty.

At the end of the ceremony, I handed out the coins, thanked everyone, and encouraged ongoing collaboration. Then I found Pat

Worsham, and we walked down the hallway to Lieutenant Colonel Demmin's office.

When I sat down, Lieutenant Colonel Demmin caught me by surprise. She said that Bruce Ivins had been "acting strange" that day and made some "strange remarks" during a therapy session. She believed that Bruce's son had called the police, afraid that Bruce was a suicide risk. The local police escorted him from USAMRIID for a medical evaluation. Now I understood why Bruce had left the celebration early.

It was now seven years after the 2001 anthrax letter attacks, which had sickened twenty-two people and killed five. The ongoing FBI investigation was gathering momentum. The FBI had initially named Dr. Steven Hatfill, a physician and former USAMRIID scientist, a "person of interest," convinced he was the perpetrator, but after he fought back and held a national press conference in August 2002 declaring his innocence, the FBI backed off.

The investigation started to take a different turn around 2004. Bacteriology colleague Hank Heine recalls doing some anthrax experiments with mice. After exposing them to anthrax spores, he grew his usual cultures of the organism. He subsequently told me, "Guess what I'm seeing. I'm seeing the morphs"–the different gray or yellowish tinged colony morphologies on the red agar plates that he thought were contaminants back in 2001 from the anthrax letter that was sent to Senator Daschle. He told the FBI, "Look, I don't know what it means, but I'm working with this stuff, and it looks just like the stuff from the letters." He believes that led to renewed focus on USAMRIID personnel as potential suspects for sending the anthrax letters.

A couple of years earlier, the NIH and the DoD wanted a well-characterized "standardized" preparation of anthrax spores that could be used to test the effectiveness of new anthrax vaccines in animals. This would ensure that the spore "prep" caused consistent animal disease for comparing across experiments, so it was created by mixing multiple different cultures of anthrax. The end result was a source of concentrated spores suspended in liquid in a flask labeled Reference Material Record (RMR) 1029. The origin of the bacteria Hank used for his mouse study came from RMR-1029–from inside the Bacteriology Division. The caretaker of that flask? Bruce Ivins.

Bruce was well regarded as a brilliant anthrax scientist, but his colleagues in the institute knew him affectionately as an "extroverted introvert" or "like your quirky uncle," a juggler, Red Cross volunteer, church choir singer, and banjo player who "could be and was the life of the party a lot of times," according to colleague Hank Heine. When Hank first arrived as a new scientist at USAMRIID, Bruce welcomed him warmly, saying, "Whatever you need, I'm here to help you out."

I did not know Bruce beyond a friendly nod in the hall, but my colleagues who knew him well strongly defended his innocence. Nevertheless, the FBI began to put the squeeze on Bruce the way they had Dr. Hatfill. Bruce believed he was under constant surveillance. Hank says, "Any time he would come out in the yard, whoever was in that house [next door], usually it was a woman, would come out, kinda hang around the yard while he was out, and when he'd go back in, she'd go back in. And he noticed something in her jeans that could've been a radio or a gun, or something." The Bacteriology Division personnel were a collegial group, frequently hanging out together after work for beers on the porch of the Community Activity Center (CAC) on base, which was just across the street and base fence from Bruce's house. "There were times on nice days we were out back on that porch and you could see someone in that upper window [next door to Bruce's house] watching us," Hank told me.

Unlike Steven Hatfill, who came out swinging, Bruce began to unravel. The FBI put on more pressure. Bit by bit, as Bruce fell under more scrutiny, things snowballed. He lost his access to research and work in the containment suites. Colleague and division chief Pat Worsham said, "The FBI had been pressuring him [Bruce] more and more and it was obvious that they were, I think, trying to break him."

Bruce left town for a week on a cruise with his brother and nephew and was feeling a bit better. When he returned, he recounted his experience to some friends, and he mentioned that two attractive women on the cruise were hanging around him a lot. "I don't know why they were paying so much attention to me," Bruce said to Pat and others, but he seemed flattered.

Hank piped in and burst his bubble, "Bruce, think about it. Those two were probably FBI agents." Bruce later apparently looked up their names and came back saying, "Oh my God, you guys were right."

Bruce shared with Hank some other disturbing treatment by the FBI. In November 2007 Hank said, the FBI "came in and grabbed him and his family out of the house, took them down to [a motel] down the street, kinda divided them up. They had Andy [his teenage son] in a separate room, and they told him that if he would go ahead and turn his father in, they'd give him a sports car." A couple of friends later verified the story with Bruce's son. Pat Worsham notes that "at one point, the FBI raided his house and his office and everything and everyone that had anything to do with him. He was so shaken after that point." Another time his wife and teenage daughter were at the local mall, and an agent accosted them and said, "You know, your husband, your father killed five people." That really upset Bruce.

So at the time of our celebration of the plague vaccine, we were aware that Bruce wasn't doing well, but we hadn't heard about any concerning behavior. When Bret Purcell dropped by my office later that afternoon, he said he was baffled why the local police had treated Bruce belligerently while escorting him to their vehicle, warning him repeatedly that they would cuff him if he made any wrong moves, because Bret observed that Bruce had cooperated. That sounded like harsher treatment than someone being led away as a suicide risk should receive.

I caught up with Pat Worsham in her office again a little later that day. I asked her if the FBI's goal was to harass Bruce until he killed himself. She had raised this very same concern with Bruce because she and others in the division were worried about him. She told him that if he killed himself, he would never be able to clear his name. She also asked him once, "Bruce, you're not going to do anything stupid, are you?"

Bruce responded, "I told my daughter I would not kill myself."

At the time, it sounded like Bruce's admission to an inpatient facility would be good for him because he needed help urgently.

Bruce had been eligible to retire for years, but he enjoyed the camaraderie of his colleagues in the Bacteriology Division and kept working. On the morning of the day he was escorted out of USAM-

RIID, Bruce had announced to everyone that he was retiring. Hank Heine said, "He was on cloud 9, because he'd made a decision, he was done with this, he was going to walk away from it and everything else and they came in and then grabbed him." Bruce went "from cloud 9 to hell . . . when they took him out of there, he was broken."

Jeff Adamovicz, deputy chief of the Bacteriology Division, spoke with Bruce a couple of days later: "He was pretty despondent; he was embarrassed obviously. . . . I just thought, 'okay, this is really bad.'" He then asked Bruce, "Do you have a lawyer? You need to do just what Steven Hatfill did, you need to be aggressive, your lawyer needs to be aggressive with them, you need to fight back because, again, if you don't fight back you look guilty."

Pat Worsham also spoke to him at that time. Bruce was upset that he had been cut off from everything that had been an outlet for him for many years. He told her it was not in his nature to hurt people. "He was very concerned about what we thought," she said, "because the FBI was systematically trying to destroy every piece of strength that he had: his family, they were trying to come between him and his family, his friends, his career." It was important for him to know that others didn't believe he was capable of doing such a horrible thing.

Two days later, on Saturday morning, I planned to head into the institute early to check on monkeys in the containment lab. Before I left home, I noticed some email messages from the commander that he sent between 6:00 and 6:30 that morning. That seemed a bit odd and early for a Saturday, but I figured he was just catching up from the prior week.

As I entered the back entrance of the building, one of the security guards told me I couldn't go to the lab by the usual route. I asked him why, and he just shrugged his shoulders. I noticed yellow "DO NOT CROSS LINE" tape strung across the central corridor, so I took a detour around a series of side hallways instead.

I suspected that the FBI had put the tape up as part of one of its many visits for evidence collection. Bruce's office was located inside the cordoned off area. I decided to drop by the headquarters before entering the lab to see what was up, and I found the commander at his desk, looking fatigued and stressed. He had been contacted by the FBI at the crack of dawn requesting a short suspense visit to USAMRIID that morning.

I asked him the same question I had asked Pat Worsham, "Is this their plan—to keep harassing him [Bruce] until he kills himself?"

Sadly, at the time, I didn't know how prescient that statement was.

19

Suspicion

....

For the most part, I enjoyed the deputy commander role and the opportunity to make operational and strategic decisions that benefited the institute. I tried to protect the scientists from administrative hassles, so they could focus on science. My daily routine involved overseeing department budgets, chairing the research committee, dogging the division chiefs to prepare for our next select agent inspection, personnel issues, regular tours and briefings for high-profile visitors, and dealing with the occasional lab exposure.

My corner office in the headquarters was next to the chief scientist and director of administration and a heartbeat away from the commander's office. A nice floor-to-ceiling window and conference table gave me a spot to gaze outside and collect my thoughts as I wrestled with the daily grind and occasional crisis.

Around 4:30 p.m. a deadly silence settles over the USAMRIID headquarters. The secretaries have left for the day. The phone stops ringing, and the sounds of email typing or chatting in the foyer dies down. Most meetings have ended, so it's a chance to sign research approvals and travel requests and catch up on email. That would not happen today.

I usually left my office door open, unless I was in a meeting, so the institute personnel felt welcome to bring me their problems at any time. Most people just walked in, but this late Thursday afternoon, several days after the FBI's Saturday-morning visit, I heard a male voice call out from the foyer outside my door: "Is anyone here?"

I got up from my desk and went to the door.

In the foyer I was surprised to see one of our former USAMRIID security guards whom I had not seen for years. He now wore a Fort Detrick police uniform.

He handed me a single sheet of white paper with a BOLO, "be on the look out," message.

As I read the note, I felt my energy drain, and my vision seemed veiled by a black-and-white filter, as in a dream state. Could this really be happening?

A picture of Bruce Ivins was displayed at the top of the BOLO, an amateurish-looking xeroxed page that any high school student could generate. I had to reread the note a couple of times for it to sink in: *The individual has threatened a co-worker and should be considered armed and dangerous.*

What the hell?!

I felt sick. Although we knew that the FBI had trained its sights on Bruce as a potential suspect in the anthrax letter attacks, having this quirky guy labeled as "armed and dangerous" didn't make sense.

"Is this a joke?" I asked.

"No sir," the officer responded and shook his head. "I can't believe it myself. I've known Dr. Ivins for seven years, and I can't believe it."

"This is crazy!" I said. "I haven't heard about any threats. We need to inform the commander."

We walked across the headquarters foyer to the commander's office.

The commander's office door was closed, but he usually swung by before going home, and it was too early for him to leave. I thought I heard voices behind the door, so I knocked. He was in the office with Bret Purcell, from the Bacteriology Division.

Bret had dropped by my office earlier that afternoon to tell me that Bruce was still in the hospital, and that his serotonin levels were "sky high." He said that Bruce's antidepressant medications had to be adjusted as a result, which could explain why he had been acting strange. He felt much better now.

When the door opened, I sensed that the two of them had been discussing the same medication issue. The commander said he had just heard about the BOLO, but he hadn't seen it yet. The officer left him a copy and took another one to hand off to the USAMRIID security guards.

I told the commander and Bret that if the BOLO was linked to a real event, it was hard to watch someone on such a downward spiral. We knew this could not be good for Bruce. We talked about how it made us all sick to witness this tragedy unfold. Many people in the institute believed that Bruce was innocent and a convenient scapegoat. The commander even told a general officer at the Pentagon that "eight hundred people in the building" thought he was innocent.

I didn't catch up on my email until later that evening. Earlier that day our chief of security and operations had emailed me an EXSUM from the Fort Detrick provost marshal about a category 3 serious incident report (SIR), which stated that Bruce had threatened coworkers. A subsequent search of his house found a flak vest, two pistols (a Glock and a 9mm), and ammunition. Now the BOLO made more sense.

As the deputy commander, I was not privy to many of the direct interactions with the FBI. I found this frustrating—like acting in a play but not having the script. The commander sensed my frustration, and we sat down a couple of days later to discuss the situation. He told me that when he had served as the deputy commander (only one month earlier), his commander at the time served as the FBI's point of contact (POC) and kept the FBI discussions to himself. So he empathized with my frustration. However, now that he was commander, he became the FBI's POC, and he understood why the information had to stay with him. He believed it was best to continue this arrangement. He would inform me about anything I needed to know, but I should not worry about it otherwise.

"I understand," I said. I appreciated his candor, and frankly, as frustrating as it was not to be privy to all the FBI's activities, it made my job easier. My schedule was already brimming with other daily institute challenges and operations.

That same day the FBI visited the institute and retrieved thousands of bacteria samples that it had stored at USAMRIID for its anthrax investigation. I thought it sadly ironic that, on the one hand, USAMRIID provided sample storage, diagnostic support, and subject matter expertise for the FBI's investigation, but, on the other hand, our colleagues were targets themselves. As Jeff Adamovicz, my bacteriology colleague, summed it up, "You were an ally or a helper in the morning and in the afternoon, you were a suspect."

Hank Heine said that he was called in regularly for interviews with the FBI and the postal inspector. His treatment was respectful at first, because, he observed, "On the one hand they were trying to eliminate us, but at the same time they also needed us, because we were the ones that could help them." Interrogations increased in frequency, and he got the "good cop, bad cop" routine. Hank knew the FBI investigator from daily work at the institute, who "was an okay guy," but "there was one of these postal inspector guys, and he was downright nasty," Hank said.

Pat Worsham noted, "Some of the lesser [FBI] scientific staff tended to be more aggressive; some of them were overtly cruel. One of them made a point when I brought up the probability of a new USAMRIID building [to tell] me, 'You guys will never have a new building.'" Another FBI agent told Pat that she and others had to prove themselves innocent, not that the FBI had to prove anyone guilty. Pat said, "That had everyone's head spinning, but Bruce was more fragile than most." Many of the staff were under gag orders that prevented them from talking with other colleagues about their discussions with the FBI, which isolated and frustrated them.

No one was immune. Even the personnel in the Medical Division faced a revolving door of interrogations about whether Bruce had any undocumented exposures, required extra anthrax vaccine boosters, or had unusual skin lesions. After the FBI questioned the staff, along came the postal inspectors. They would ask the same questions and were very accusatory. Clinic chief Ellen Boudreau said, "It was all made-up behaviors they were trying to pull out from your descriptions, so it was very strange and repetitive and time wasting," but no one felt that he or she could turn down their interview requests. The inspectors also seemed to have too little knowledge of science, microbiology, or protective measures used in the lab to conduct such an investigation. "I just thought these were not the appropriate people to send to a scientific institute," Ellen said. The postal inspectors would ask, "Is that what you told the FBI?" as they looked for discrepancies in her testimony. When anyone would go to the USAMRIID library, the FBI agents in three-piece suits who had camped out there were "kind of eyeing you to see what you were looking at, so it was a little bit intimidating to have the FBI watching your every move," Ellen recalled.

Hank speculated, "[The FBI was] working an idea that maybe it wasn't one of us, that maybe it was a group of us or we knew somebody did it, but because they were our friend, we were trying to cover for him." They would tell Hank, "Bruce said that you did this, or Bruce said that you did that," as they tried to sow dissention and paranoia among the group, because, as Hank remarked, "You know, there's no honor among thieves."

Apparently, those tactics began to have an effect on Bruce, who believed Hank was incriminating him. The FBI came to Hank and said, "Look, we're very concerned. Bruce has made threats that he's going to do something to you and we're going to try and protect you. What do you want us to do about this?" Hanks response: "Nothing, because Bruce isn't going to do anything to me." The next day at work, the Fort Detrick police came to Hank's office and asked the same thing, "What do you want to do about this?" Hank believes they wanted him to put out a protection order. He wouldn't do it. Within forty-eight hours, though, Bruce's therapist did, which led to the BOLO. Among other things she cited a "threatening" message that Bruce had left on her phone. Curiously, the tape contained no threats, only resignation by a man whose life had been shattered, or as the *Frederick News Post* declared, "the sad ramblings of a broken man who felt betrayed."[1]

All the while many members of the Bacteriology Division were convinced that their phones were tapped. Jeff said, "I heard weird clicking noise and stuff on the phone all the time," and Hank noticed that the division's "computers every once in a while would do like somebody's taking a screen shot." Three years earlier, in February 2005, the FBI "actually came in and confiscated all our computers and mirrored the hard drives" and returned them twenty-four hours later. The group also wondered whether some lab technicians hired recently in the division were FBI infiltrators. "Either they had the place bugged, or there was somebody in our group that had infiltrated," Hank surmised, because conversations that division staff had had casually over a beer would come up in the next interview.

Pat Worsham was less convinced that her phone was tapped, saying, "It would sort of click in and out. This was a government phone, so no real surprises there." But she also noted, "They were following us; we knew they followed us; they told us we were being followed." She noticed a black SUV parked a block from her house every night for a long time. One day she went to a routine doctor's appointment, and when she came back, someone from the FBI called her and said, "I hope your health is well." "It was creepy," Pat said.

One day in the clinic, Ellen Boudreau saw the suite supervisor for one of the suites where Bruce worked. This woman sang in her church choir. She was "really upset," because the FBI had told her fellow choir members that she had some knowledge about what was going on, but she was keeping it to herself and asked them whether she was a suspicious character.

Feeling pressure from the constant scrutiny, some tried to fight back in subtle and not so subtle ways. Hank Heine had a farm in West Virginia on a ridge with surrounding ridges and valleys. He and his USAMRIID buddies would go out there a couple of times a year for target practice. They called themselves the "Bacti Militia."

"Every time we were there," Hank said, "two or three black Suburbans would come pulling out on that other ridge, and the guys would get out with binoculars and watch us." Hank exhibits a balance of cynicism and *Family Guy / South Park* sense of humor. At one point he and his buddies dropped their trousers and mooned the agents.

The next week when he was called in for questioning, the agents told him, "We didn't find that very funny." Hank played dumb and responded, "You didn't find what funny?" "You know exactly what we're talking about," they insisted. "Oh," said Hank, "you mean you guys were watching us while I was up at my farm?" Hank chuckled as he recalled the meeting, but at the time, he said, having a little gallows humor helped them all to cope.

Even more disturbing to the team, Jeff says "The FBI was bringing in people at night, and the security people were told to shut off the cameras and they were going into the suites . . . and doing God knows what. We have no idea what they were doing, but they weren't allowed to be escorted; they weren't allowed to be filmed." This news created intense paranoia—were they planting evidence, sampling peoples' work? This unsupervised activity was completely against protocol, but somehow the agents were allowed to do it.

But the most disturbing question that the investigation raised was, Where was the army? The army was completely hands off and offered no legal counsel or pushback for its own employees. Pat Worsham said, "We were talking to the grand jury, and JAG [judge advocate general, i.e., army lawyers] made it very clear that they were not there to help us in any way, that they were only there to coach us so that we didn't say anything stupid that would impact the government, basically."

Hank said, "We were under investigation because we worked there and we're doing our jobs and we were being left there out on our own."

Pat reached the sad conclusion that the army "may not have thrown us under the bus, but they saw the bus coming, and they didn't look away, and they didn't pick up the pieces after it happened. It could've been that we shouldn't have expected any help, but you try to think of the army values, you know 'loyalty' and so on and 'selfless service' and those things we have posted on the wall and I think we have a lot of people who are invested in that, but it doesn't seem to go two ways."

At the end of the day, when the FBI retrieved its samples from the investigation, the commander gave me a copy of a memorandum written to Bruce Ivins by Fort Detrick's garrison commander, who determines who can and can't enter a military base. The memo stated that Bruce was barred from entering Fort Detrick without prior authorization and an escort. I suspected this could be the final nail in the coffin for someone who had spent a couple of decades working there.

Bruce was due for discharge from the hospital the next day. The commander had called Bruce's wife earlier in the day to give her advanced warning of the memo. He had waited to see if Bruce would call back, but he hadn't. I would be acting commander for the next several days. So if Bruce called while the commander was out of town, I should convey three things to Bruce: he must have an occupational health evaluation; someone would have to escort him on base solely for the evaluation; and he would be placed on administrative leave until his pending retirement. This action was not intended to be punitive, and he would still receive pay and other entitlements until things were sorted out.

We had significant concerns that Bruce was already in a fragile state, and we didn't want to do anything that might push him over the edge. We envisioned a scenario where Bruce might drive up to Fort Detrick's entrance gate without realizing he had been barred from the post and cause a scene that would dig him deeper into trouble.

Bruce never called me back that Friday, but the commander emailed me over the weekend to let me know that he had spoken with Bruce. Unfortunately, Bruce complained of a headache and didn't want to talk, so he never received the message about being barred from post entry.

Bruce never called back again after that.

Five days later, on July 29, 2008, I attended a noon lecture by the commander at the National Cancer Institute on Fort Detrick. Afterward I asked him whether he had heard from Bruce. No, he said, but he had just learned that Bruce had been found at home, unconscious. He didn't know any more at the time.

Back at my office later that evening, around 5:15 p.m., I heard some chatter in the office of the chief scientist, Peter Hobart, next door, so I went to check it out.

The commander and Peter were commiserating, and they shared the sad news: Bruce was dead. I remember that moment clearly. As with the Kennedy assassination, most people in the institute I have spoken with since then remember where they were when they learned about Bruce's death.

The news hit me hard. I had to sit down to absorb the shock and disbelief.

We talked for a while about Bruce, and we all felt a sense of loss. The commander subsequently sent a note of condolence to the entire institute, and a chaplain came by to speak with aggrieved staff.

We later learned that Bruce had killed himself with an overdose that included acetaminophen (Tylenol), a drug that destroys the liver when taken in massive quantities.

I wondered about the implications of Bruce's death for the institute. We couldn't fully assess it at the time, but the impact would be broad and far reaching.

20

The Aftermath

··

After I returned home that evening, I sat at my desk to ponder the day's tragic news. I still couldn't believe that Bruce was dead.

From prior experience with other highly charged events, I had a good sense of what sparked media interest. I worried that once word of Bruce's death got out, all hell would break loose, and the media would descend on the institute. I fired off an email to the commander, saying we should get Caree, our public affairs officer, working on potential responses to media queries.

The next two days were quiet. I walked around the somber hallways commiserating with people, allowing them to vent, and trying to do my part to hold the institute together. Bruce's "home," in the Bacteriology Division, especially, was in mourning. On July 31, two days after Bruce's death, I spoke with several personnel in the division's front office. With teary, red eyes, the division secretary shared that Bruce had told her that the FBI harassment would end only "when I'm dead." In retrospect that was clearly a cry for help.

We frequently spoke of the "USAMRIID family," built by generations of workers who had spent their entire careers there. The sorrow of the Bacteriology Division's personnel was emblematic of the pall that crept over the entire institute. Many had felt suspicion and anger with the FBI investigation and especially the investigation of Bruce. They believed that the course of events had not needed to take such a tragic turn, and that the army should have backed up one of its own scientists. For most the idea that Bruce, our "quirky uncle" who wore rainbow-colored suspenders, would do something as heinous as sending the anthrax letters was inconceivable.

Someone must have leaked Bruce's death to the press—either the FBI or someone within the institute—because several colleagues received early-morning phone calls the next two days, on July 30 and 31, from news outlets. Hank Heine recalls a midnight call from the *Los Angeles Times*: "You work with Bruce Ivins. The Justice Department is going to announce that he is the anthrax mailer. Do you have any comments?" He responded, "I talked to the grand jury, and I can't make any comments," and hung up. Sensing a gathering storm, the next morning a group from Bacteriology met at Nallin Pond, a picturesque area on Fort Detrick nearby USAMRIID with rolling green hills, weeping willows, picnic tables, and an old barn. They wanted to get out of the institute to a place where they could be by themselves, talk privately, and avoid inviting unwanted scrutiny. They were also concerned that they didn't know who was listening or what was bugged. "We wanted to get ahead of it because we knew what was coming," Hank says. They knew Bruce would be "thrown under the bus, because he was dead," but they didn't want the media reports to dictate Bruce's memory, and they wanted to ensure that he would be treated like any other colleague who had died tragically.

"We had relied on each other for years," Pat Worsham said, "with no help from the outside. Nobody else supported us; nobody gave us moral support. We went to the people who had carried us through all along, and that was each other." The group planned memorial services for Bruce, on and off Fort Detrick. "There were people who gave little testimonials and we reminisced, and we laughed, and we cried," she recalled.

David Willman, a Pulitzer Prize–winning reporter from the *Los Angeles Times* covering the anthrax investigation, had scheduled a visit to USAMRIID for August 7. That visit never happened. Instead, he broke the story about Bruce's suicide on August 1.

The wave of media interest came crashing down even more heavily than I had predicted. The day after the story broke, a feeding frenzy vaulted the story to the front page of the *Washington Post* and other newspapers across the country. It would continue relentlessly for more days than any other USAMRIID news event I had experienced.

We issued a press release. In addition, Caree asked me whether we should release a photo of Bruce, because news outlets were asking for one. We debated the benefits and the downside of doing so, but decided to release a photo of Bruce wearing a formal jacket and tie with a boutonnière. I thought his lopsided, tentative smile and sad eyes in the photo ironically fitting for the occasion. Numerous other photos eventually made it into the newspapers: images of Bruce as a Red Cross volunteer, receiving an award for his research, and juggling.

I caught up with a frazzled institute commander at the end of the day. He wasn't getting much support from the army higher-ups, who seemed to be distancing themselves; however, he did receive a nice note from the army surgeon general, who expressed condolences and concern for the well-being of the Ivins family.

I had to leave town on August 2 for a previously scheduled trip. I felt guilty leaving after this bombshell had dropped, but the commander encouraged me to go anyway. Before I left, we discussed the possibility of submitting a memo of formal protest to the army surgeon general about the way the investigation had treated our personnel and the FBI's methods used to "squeeze" Bruce.

While I was out of town, I watched the news feeds in the evening, and the news content at that time appeared balanced, noting why Bruce was under suspicion, but also included his scientific achievements and endearing quirks. The institute held a memorial service at Fort Detrick for friends and colleagues on base, attended by hundreds. Afterward a couple of colleagues were toasting Bruce's memory at a bar, when the anthrax story appeared on TV. They were all shouting at the TV, which upset some people around them, and one of the bacteriology group nearly got into a fight.

I returned the following Saturday, August 9, 2008, in time to attend a second, larger memorial service for Bruce at his church in downtown Frederick, Maryland. The bright sun cast shadows across the cobblestone sidewalks as I walked briskly down the narrow streets to St. John the Evangelist Roman Catholic Church. Three days earlier the FBI had named Bruce as the anthrax letter mailer. They cited his access to the presumed anthrax source (Flask RMR-1029), his knowledge of spore-growing techniques, long hours spent in the lab around the time of the attacks in 2001, a presumed attempt to throw the FBI off his trail based on an incorrect sample he submitted to them, and a history of psychological problems and odd behaviors. So I wasn't surprised to see a group of reporters camped out across the street from the church, with some speaking into microphones in front of camera tripods.

The large chapel was packed. I squeezed into a pew near the front just before the service began. One by one Bruce's colleagues, friends, and family came to the pulpit to speak. Bret Purcell, a Bacteriology coworker, summarized Bruce's scientific achievements, and Pat Worsham, Bacteriology Division chief, provided more personal anecdotes about his endearing quirks, pranks, and comedic moments.[1]

Genuine love, sadness, and a chorus of sniffles surrounded me in the chapel, as friends, colleagues, and family members dabbed their eyes. I thought to myself, *This doesn't seem like the funeral of a murderer.* The reception afterward had a touching display of Bruce's family photos from various stages of his life and a complete bibliography of his scientific publications.

Pat Worsham met a man at the reception who claimed to be a fellow parishioner but then started peppering her with questions. When she noticed him writing down her answers, she realized he was a reporter. She berated him, telling him that he needed to leave immediately or she would call someone to escort him out. He was not the only mole in the crowd, because I recognized many quotations from the service in the press the next day.

The institute had been in the FBI's crosshairs for seven years, but the naming of Bruce as the anthrax perpetrator brought the most heat thus far. The commander and a DoD undersecretary had discussed a potential strategy to counter some of the bad press. Two days after the funeral, at our routine Monday-morning headquarters meeting, the commander informed us that the secretary of the army had visited him the week prior, while I was away. During that meeting the commander had raised his concerns and counterarguments about the FBI's case, including objecting to the treatment of our personnel and Bruce's family during the investigation. The secretary told him forcefully that the army would make *no objection* to the

The Aftermath

FBI case and would focus its efforts on moving forward. The army preferred to emphasize the changes that had already been implemented to USAMRIID's program.

The commander told us, "I probably made my one mistake [as a commander]." The next one would cost him his job. That bothered me, but I was not surprised. I had been around long enough to know that the army would protect its interests and try to move on. The Pentagon expends enough energy regularly dodging alligators. The last thing the leadership would want was finger-pointing between different branches of government (Defense and Justice), but the FBI investigation was the mother of all public relations nightmares. It was probably good that I had missed the meeting with the secretary. I might have pressed the point and become the sacrificial lamb.

USAMRIID has numerous visiting congressmen and senators, who swing by regularly in limos or helicopters to watch laboratory personnel working in space suits, because they read about it in *The Hot Zone*. It all makes for a good "dog and pony" show. On August 15 the army surgeon general and Fort Detrick's commanding general visited USAMRIID together, but for a significantly different purpose. The surgeon general had "walked the halls" before as our prior commanding general. Even so the frequency of his visits during this period was unprecedented. In my ten years associated with USAMRIID at the time, I had seen only one surgeon general visit for a few minutes. The visit by the secretary of the army *and* the army surgeon general in quick succession demonstrated how serious the Pentagon considered the Ivins affair.

The institute held a series of town-hall meetings, so the two generals could address the entire workforce. The surgeon general opened by expressing condolences for the loss of Bruce and the tainting of the institute. He likened the events surrounding the anthrax letters and suspicion cast on USAMRIID to the institute's "own 9/11." Similar to what happened to the country after 9/11, we couldn't go back to the previous state of affairs.

He demonstrated amazing perception and empathy, recognizing the institute's profound loss of one of its own, even while acknowledging the FBI's grave accusations against Bruce.

Then he spoke about the future. The army would do what it knows best: it would set up a defensive perimeter to protect the institute. The Pentagon would form a task force, led by a two-star general, to develop new policies for managing the bioweapon agents in our inventory. This task force would serve as the "tip of the spear" for anything related to the anthrax attacks, including dealing with the press.

Although the visiting generals tried to reassure the assembled USAMRIID workforce, anyone who has dealt with the army bureaucracy knows that when they hear, "We're from the army and we're here to help," it is time to duck for cover.

The mood in the audience reflected concern that our already-diminished autonomy to do science would be restricted further. The army would get into all aspects of our business—down to everyone's underwear brand name, size, and color. We were assured that the task force would need our help to reform our threat agent policies, but the staff greeted this notion with significant skepticism. We anticipated further "punishment" on the horizon.

We had reason to be skeptical. We had heard the same after 9/11 and the anthrax attacks, when many policies changed. So the army could have chosen a different tack to trumpet the significant changes we had made already over the previous seven years. Instead it decided to do one better. The task force issued numerous new policies that would further burden the already-reeling institute. As virology technician Dianne Negley complained, people "who didn't understand science, who didn't know how to work on this stuff put new regulations on that were not for our best safety. . . . You're causing the possibility of another accident. You're increasing it instead of decreasing it."

Four days later I received a short-notice request from our commanding general's headquarters office across Fort Detrick to bring everyone there immediately who had been involved in Bruce's laboratory clearance. I made a couple of quick phone calls and emails to pull the relevant people together. Before the meeting we sat down and drafted key points about the differences in how we conducted operations before versus after 9/11.

We learned that the general had been "asked" (I suspected ordered) by the Pentagon's task force to do an interview with a reporter from USA Today who planned to write a negative editorial about the institute. I was surprised, and wondered, *Wasn't that the task force's job, to provide top cover with the press?*

A group of us, including the USAMRIID commander; Bret Purcell, the general's chief of staff; the public affairs officers from USAMRIID and from the general's staff; and me, met with the general to help prepare him for his interview. I had concerns about the interview because I had witnessed how a prior commander was mishandled by the press.

At the end of the meeting, I told the general, "I am afraid this is a set-up."

He tilted his head and with a resigned shrug responded, "Welcome to my world."

After the meeting I cornered the two public affairs officers in the hallway and asked why the task force had changed its ground rules. And why was the task force so anxious now to respond to the press, when it had not done so previously? They didn't know, but they said they would bring up my concerns with the general.

As we left the building, I shared with my colleagues my concerns that I feared the Pentagon wanted a military face associated with the crisis, and it might be setting the general up for a fall.

Fortunately, the interview went well. USA Today printed a counter-editorial by our general, which was far better than any of us could have hoped for. I am happy to report that my fears weren't realized.

A year and a half after Bruce's death, the FBI formally closed the anthrax case with the conclusion that Bruce Ivins was the sole perpetrator of the anthrax attacks.

To this day his closest colleagues believe Bruce was innocent—a convenient patsy in a high-profile case that the FBI was under tremendous pressure to solve. Had the FBI decided that Bruce was the killer and ignored any evidence that did not fit with its hypothesis, rather than try to understand and explain the pieces that didn't fit? Although Bruce conducted significant research on anthrax and the anthrax vaccine during his thirty-six-year career (eighteen of those years at USAMRIID), some of the nation's top biodefense experts have questioned whether he had the skill set to create the form of anthrax found in the letters. Hank Heine asserts, "First and foremost, despite what everybody says, he actually didn't have the knowledge to produce the material the way it was in those envelopes." Jeff Adamovicz claims that the spores in the letters "contain[ed] high levels of silica and tin" and cites a 2011 scientific paper by anthrax experts that pointed to "a high degree of manufacturing skill, contrary to reassurances that the attack germs were unsophisticated," although others thought that the tin could have been a random contaminant.[2] Jeff suggests that the FBI "supposedly tried to re-create the spores using equipment Bruce had access to, using the time frame in which they speculated he did it, and they couldn't re-create that material." The FBI never explained the origin of another organism found in one of the letters, *Bacillus subtilis niger*. The agency couldn't locate it in his laboratory or in RMR-1029. Furthermore, Jeff notes, they "found no physical evidence, despite extensive searches of his home, his cars, his mailboxes, his laboratory."

Graduating from a liquid slurry to the dried powder in the letters would be a significant engineering leap for a microbiologist. It takes more than just putting it in a dryer to prevent clumping and binding to other particles in the environment, and the average Joe would be hard pressed to do so in his bathtub or garage. What is more, the spores in the letter were exponentially smaller—and therefore more concentrated per given amount—than anything created by the U.S. or Soviet bioweapons programs over decades. The dryer that Bruce was presumed to have used, a lyophilizer kept in a nearby hallway, was broken. Pat Worsham doesn't believe it was physically possible to generate the spores inside USAMRIID. She explains, "The lyophilizer we had in the Division at the time was on the cold side; it was extremely heavy. If he [Bruce] was going to take that in containment he would've had to get help to put it in the airlock and get it out and run a decon, which we did not do ourselves, and take it back out." Hank says, even if it had worked and Bruce had pulled it into the lab, "it has no filter on it, and in the process of drying those spores down, it would have sucked spores into the whole instrument and . . . some of them would have gotten blown back out through the vacuum source," causing a massive contamination. The FBI "tore it all apart and looked for anthrax DNA and they found nothing," Jeff concludes.

Hank also argues that although the FBI claimed Bruce was working long hours in the lab immediately after 9/11, Bruce commonly worked long and late hours, and everyone knew that was his normal pattern. Furthermore, right after 9/11 Fort Detrick went under Threatcon Delta. Full lockdown. It was hard to get on base. Hank was stuck overseas for a week. "Bruce, living right there, could walk up and get in and was doing everyone's animal checks," for their experiments, including his own. "Bruce was kinda taking care of everybody's stuff. When did Bruce have time to grow up and harvest anthrax, turning anthrax into powder?" Hank asks.

Hank believes it would have taken Bruce nine months or more to produce the number of spores in the letters, not the few weeks around 9/11 when the FBI presumed he did. Using basic algebra he argues that to fill about 2 grams of anthrax powder in each letter at a concentration of 10^{12} spores per gram, and multiplied by 5 letters would require 10^{13} (10 trillion) spores. "The yield for a spore run is 10^8 (100 million) under the best of conditions." That is multiple orders of magnitude to scale up—a difference of 100,000 times, which translates to 100 to 200 liters of anthrax fermenting. Such a large-scale operation would be hard to hide from coworkers and avoid contaminating the lab. Pat Worsham says, "The fact that some of those morphs were in RMR-1029 I think is a clue, but it is not proof that it came from here because a lot of spores in that prep came from Dugway [Proving Ground].[3] And they were running fermenters [at Dugway]. And I have not seen those kinds of morphs in our spore preparations. . . . We worked with flasks, so that's small volume, relatively, compared to fermenter runs. That's why we got Dugway to make spores for us, because it was hard to make enough."

Despite the FBI's conclusions, and the portrait painted by the FBI and in the media of Bruce as a gun-toting, homicidal sociopath who cross-dressed and obsessed about a woman's sorority, Bruce's coworkers held a very different view of the man. Hank says the final piece is Bruce himself. He was a devout Catholic. Even if Bruce came up with some strange justification to do this to give the country a wake-up call or for some other reason, Hank says, "As soon as he realized that people actually died as a result of it, I don't think he could have lived with himself, let alone sit there and hang out with everybody for eight more years. That's the Bruce I knew and know." Jeff Adamovicz agrees: "I don't think he had the moral fortitude to do it. I think you have to have a certain amount of hatred in your personality to pull something like this off, and I don't think he had that. He volunteered for the Red Cross; he juggled; he sang at church choir. . . . He wasn't an aggressive person."

Paul F. Kemp, Bruce's attorney, called the investigation "an orchestrated dance of carefully worded statements, heaps of innuendo, and a staggering lack of real evidence" that appeared to have been successful in its objective.[4] Bruce Ivins is dead, so we will never know his side of the story, which has left his colleagues frustrated that there was no trial, where both perspectives might have been heard.

Some have said that because Bruce committed suicide, he must have been guilty, but it isn't hard to see what could have driven Bruce to suicide. His downward spiral took many turns, as piece by piece his connection to his livelihood and coworkers unraveled. He faced legal bills in the hundreds of thousands of dollars. And after he had worked thirty-plus years for the government on defenses against anthrax, the FBI planned to seek the death penalty. All this could seem like the ultimate betrayal and might easily push someone *on* the edge *over* the edge.

One of the bedrocks of the U.S. democracy, that someone is innocent until proven guilty in a court of law, seems to have been ignored. As one colleague noted, there is "no such thing as guilty by suicide."

Sadly, this story has no happy ending. Twenty-two individuals became infected with anthrax from tainted letters, and five of them died. Dr. Stephen Hatfill, the FBI's first "person of interest," was eventually exonerated. Although he received a $5.8 million settlement, his life and career had been shattered. Dr. Bruce Ivins died from his own hand.

After his death four of his colleagues, all anthrax experts, wrote a tribute to Bruce in the scientific journal *Microbe*.[5] In addition to citing his long history of scientific accomplishments, they noted that he was "an enthusiastic teacher, coworker, and mentor to his technicians, students, and colleagues . . . a skilled poet, songwriter, and musician; a dedicated volunteer. . . . His colleagues and friends will remember him not only for his dedication to his work, but also for his humor, curiosity, and great generosity."

Getting those four scientific rivals to agree on anything was an accomplishment in and of itself.

Since Bruce's death, the handling of the anthrax case has been questioned by several government authorities and other agencies. Senator Patrick Leahy expressed skepticism that Ivins acted alone when hearing testimony from FBI Director Robert Mueller in committee hearings. A National Academy of Science committee concluded that it was "impossible to reach any definitive conclusion about the origins of the anthrax in the letters, based solely on the available scientific evidence." The report also challenged the FBI and the U.S. Justice Department's conclusion that a single-spore batch of anthrax maintained by Ivins in his laboratory at Fort Detrick was the parent material for the spores in the anthrax letters. Even different branches of the Justice Department appeared to have trouble deciding what to believe, as its own civil attorneys "contradicted their own department's conclusion that Ivins was unquestionably the anthrax killer" when filing their motions to defend the government against a civil case brought by the family of the first victim (Robert Stevens).[6] The case was settled out of court.

The scientific debate will continue; however, vindication for Bruce Ivins seems far off, although in a bizarre twist, a former FBI agent who led the anthrax investigation for four years, is suing his former agency, stating there is "a staggering amount of exculpatory evidence" that the FBI has yet to reveal. He accuses the FBI of trying "to railroad the prosecution" and bolster its claim of Ivins's guilt after his death.[7]

Dr. Vahid Majidi, chief scientist for the FBI's anthrax investigation, wrote a book titled *A Spore on the Grassy Knoll: An Insider's Account of the 2001 Anthrax Mailings*, which implies that Bruce's innocence or guilt will not be resolved to everyone's satisfaction. It will remain, like the Kennedy assassination, shrouded in "what ifs" and potential conspiracy theories for decades. Only God knows the truth about what happened and whether Bruce Ivins really perpetrated the anthrax attacks. Unfortunately, the negative impact of the investigation on the institute continues to this day. Some scientists, fed up with the regulations that the army and other agencies ratcheted up in the aftermath, voted with their feet.

The army has routine requirements for employees to watch training videos on espionage and terrorism defense. To add insult to injury, alongside a host of spies who had sold out to the Russians or other foreign countries, one year the videos included Bruce Ivins as an example of suspicious characters to be on the lookout for. Many colleagues were outraged when they saw it.

Not everyone believes as strongly as Bruce's colleagues Hank Heine, Jeff Adamovicz, and Pat Worsham that Bruce could not have sent the letters. Some are more equivocal, stating that they "didn't know then and don't know now," whether Bruce could have done it. There may be others in the institute who agree with the FBI's conclusion, but they have been less vocal. However, eleven years after his death, several of his closest colleagues remain defiant.

Pat Worsham says now, "I think we were bitter. I think we still are bitter, angry, that it went down the way it did. I think that the FBI knew how hard they'd been pushing him, that he had psychological issues, and they were hitting all the buttons that they could possibly hit."

Hank Heine says, "I'll go to my grave believing Bruce had nothing to do with it."

If you walk down the narrow hallway next to the Bacteriology Division offices at USAMRIID today, you will pass a locked glass case on the wall for displaying awards received by division members. There are only three awards currently in the display case. The one defiantly at dead center is a medal and certificate for "Exceptional Civilian Service" to the government. The name on the award: Bruce Ivins.

21

Down for the Count

How easy is it to get anthrax, plague, Ebola samples?

It turns out, not that difficult. Prior to the 1990–91 "first" Gulf War (Operation Desert Storm), the United States suspected that Iraq had a robust biological warfare program. After the war Iraq admitted to weaponizing 10,000 liters of botulinum toxin and 6,500 liters of anthrax. The country wasn't fooling around.

The big surprise, though, was that Iraq obtained one of its seed strains to make anthrax and botulinum toxins through legal means from a culture collection in the United States, a microbe "warehouse" for legitimate research and medical purposes.[1] Similar microbe collections exist around the world that ship and sell deadly pathogens, including the Chessmen. How Iraq got them is now apparent, but it showed that a determined adversary could obtain the top six threat agents at will.

Move ahead to 1995. Microbiologist and former white supremacist Larry Wayne Harris was caught with *Yersinia pestis*, the bacteria that causes plague, in his glove compartment.

Question: where did he get it?

Answer: from the same U.S. culture collection as Iraq.

The laws for bioterrorism were in their infancy, so he was convicted, not for possessing plague but for mail fraud, because he had misrepresented himself on paperwork when ordering it.

Since then the laws have tightened significantly. Now anyone who wants to work with the Chessmen and any other select agents in the United States must register with the CDC. Shipments of the pathogens are tracked closely, with much more stringent procedures and in some cases require an armed escort. Select agents are pathogens determined by the government to have the "potential to pose a severe threat to both human and animal health, to plant health, or to animal and plant products."[2] As a result there are specific requirements for handling, storing, and shipping them.

During the year I served as USAMRIID's deputy commander, we were constantly pedaling to keep up with the changing government rules on managing select agents.[3]

Throughout USAMRIID we had seventy thousand vials of select agents, scattered across nearly six hundred freezers and refrigerators in the BSL-2, BSL-3, and BSL-4 labs. Each minus-eighty-degree freezer has four to five drawers or cabinets caked with one-half-inch-thick frost, which could easily hide a stray vial. The vials are tiny, less than an inch to perhaps two inches tall, and are kept inside multiple individual boxes. The number of vials was a constant moving target, because with each experiment, new vials of organisms or tissue might be created or destroyed.

Every batch of select agents in the institute had to be under the authority of a single scientist or technician who kept track of how much he or she had in storage at all times. In the past it wasn't a major issue. The agents were kept in storage in freezers inside the containment labs. The high hurdles, multiple barriers, and lengthy training time it took to gain lab access provided a strong firewall against anyone intent on stealing agents. But as the rules changed, the individual accountability for owning and tracking the agents became more onerous and riskier.

The army instituted a new program called the Personnel Reliability Program (PRP) to investigate and scrutinize people before they entered a containment lab to ensure that they weren't criminals, didn't use drugs, or have a disqualifying medical issue. Personnel had to report any changes in their health status, prescription medications, and dental treatments. We probably had the largest number of people in a single institute working on these agents on the planet, at over two hundred individuals. In the aftermath of Bruce Ivins's death, we were under intense pressure by the army inspector general (IG) to comply with the new rules. In 2007, in true Army fashion, we were given only a couple of months to get 100 percent of the workers enrolled in the PRP; otherwise the army surgeon general would shut us down.

At any given time, we were preparing for an inspection, being inspected, or responding to inspection findings from multiple organizations. Rather than killing us with one thousand little cuts, it felt more like multiple body blows. At one point we felt so pummeled that we started wondering whether there was a conspiracy to shut us down. Our operations team was drowning in paperwork responding to the inspections, and our scientists were frustrated by all the delays the inspections caused in keeping their essential research on track. One inspection was particularly galling. At the end of a CDC evaluation, during their outbrief the inspectors said that we should expect only about a dozen "findings" to address. We briefed our commanding general on the good news. But when the report came out, the CDC listed ninety-three findings. It had cited the same finding repeatedly for each one of our containment laboratories, thus multiplying the findings eightfold. We felt betrayed.

Our lead for operations, Lieutenant Colonel Dave Shoemaker, oversaw our agent accountability and inspection responses. Although Dave had a softer side, and he loved nothing more than hanging out on his sailboat, his shaved head and ramrod military bearing jibed with his meticulous compulsiveness. He had the right personality for the job, and I trusted him implicitly. Dave was particularly incensed by the CDC's bait and switch. When he finally finished addressing all the findings, as a subtle way to express his displeasure, Dave sent the CDC a shipment of nineteen three-ring binders, which included three versions of the relevant documents: the original version, versions showing tracked changes, and new, revised documents. Years later when he learned that the CDC's lead inspector was angry to receive such a voluminous response, Dave smiled to himself.

The PRP extended to agent accountability. Someone who didn't manage his or her inventory properly could be deemed "unreliable" and blocked from lab entry. Not surprisingly some scientists preferred to avoid taking on that risk.

In 2008 one long-term USAMRIID scientist left the institute for a job elsewhere, so another scientist had to pick up his agents. The receiving investigator compared the agent list she inherited with the actual vials in the lab freezers.

One afternoon I learned that three vials of VEE on the list were missing. *Oh shit!* I thought. What happened to them? In natural outbreaks in Central and South America, mosquitoes spread VEE among horses, which kills them. But VEE can also infect through the air. It is considered a "reliable" weapon because it sickens nearly 100 percent of the people who inhale it. Most other viruses aren't as efficient. The virus grows and replicates in the brain and surrounding fluids, causing high fevers, body aches, and an excruciating headache. Victims don't usually die, but they might wish they were dead; they may stay in bed for a week or two. The risk to a military operation is obvious because it's hard to drive a tank or dig a foxhole if you feel like you've been run over by a truck. A terrorist could spray enough of it over a city to knock down hundreds to thousands of people.

When we queried the departing investigator about the inventory mismatch, he believed that the missing vials had been used up and discarded after experiments by someone else years ago, but the paperwork had failed to catch up. He had never even worked on VEE and probably inherited the list of vials from someone else. Our internal assessment concurred. We sent the requisite EXSUM up the chain, stating, "A thorough internal USAMRIID investigation concluded that past accounting errors of this large inventory was responsible for this discrepancy." In the past this would have been the end of it—but not in the current climate.

The army uses SIRs to notify the Pentagon about major disasters, like a soldier's death or a helicopter crash. A missing vial qualified as an SIR, which Dave Shoemaker dutifully fired off. This triggered alarm bells around the Washington, DC Beltway. The Criminal Investigation Division (CID), the military version of the FBI, paid us a visit. You don't want to tangle with these people—they have no sense of humor.

Before launching their investigation, the lead CID investigator sat down with Dave Shoemaker to agree on some ground rules "for nonconfrontational conversation, not heavy hitting," Dave said. "Questioning of RIID folks was not going to be a hardcore 'good cop/bad cop' type scenario, but simply information gathering."

That's not what happened, however. If you are a hammer, everything is a nail. If you are a CID investigator, everyone is a criminal, even when none exist. When the CID started interviewing USAMRIID staff, "It was totally the opposite of what I had been led to believe," Dave said. At least a half dozen people came to him upset—some on the verge of tears, feeling "like they were criminal suspects." This was particularly frightening for the workers in the post-anthrax investigation climate. This "lit my fuse," Dave related, and he had some heated exchanges with the CID.

Nonetheless, the investigation continued for five months . . . involving thirty special agents conducting over five hundred interviews and documenting 1,250 man-hours on a wild-goose chase over *five continents* at a cost of $500,000. The CID concluded that it was probably a clerical error left over from decades prior. Hmm. Didn't we conclude that five months earlier . . . for free? I shared Dave's concern that "this was an incredible waste of time, money, and resources." The departing scientist felt that after years of dedicated service, he was an easy target for blame, because he had already left the institute. It all seemed a bit of overkill, but after 9/11 and the anthrax attacks, the environment was heavily charged.

Dave considered the VEE investigation "growing pains," as we transitioned our mind-set away from the days when a scientist could carry a "VIP" (vial in pocket) of a disease agent or a patient sample when returning from a foreign country. The take-home lesson for me was that scientists could now go to jail merely for a clerical error.

That was the fate of Dr. Tom Butler, a Vietnam veteran, highly respected plague expert, and infectious disease professor in Texas. In 2003 he reported a discrepancy in his plague sample numbers, as would be required under the new rules. Instead of being applauded, he was accused of bioterrorism. He was eventually exonerated for bioterrorism, but the investigation dug up financial irregularities from his research grants. He spent two years in a penitentiary and lost his medical license, despite outcries from respected medical societies and colleagues.[4] We were in a new world order.

Inventory scrutiny dogged us like a toothache with the occasional root canal. Dave says, "I lost more nights' sleep for that than anything else." At one point the USAMRIID commander confided to him that he wrote in his daily log book, "I will get fired today," after a tough meeting with our commanding general. Dave subsequently told me that the inventory issues might be enough for the Pentagon's anthrax response task force to shut down the institute or to relieve the commander. I told Dave, "If the commander goes, I'm going with him." Dave said he would too. Dave went home that evening and broke down, feeling guilty that an inventory error could sack "the best commander [he] had ever served under."

We were already reeling from the emotional toll of constant scrutiny.

Then the next shoe dropped.

On February 4, 2009, I walked into Dave's office next to the USAMRIID headquarters. Given his job responsibilities, Dave usually had a humorless demeanor, but I could occasionally get him to crack a smile—not today. Dave was with one of his Operations Section chiefs. They told me that an army inspector that day had inventoried a list of sixteen vials of VEE in the freezer.

They found twenty vials instead—another inventory mismatch.

Damn. Feeling a familiar punch in the gut, I had to sit down. I understood the implications immediately. Not only was this on the heels of the missing VEE vials, but over a year earlier, the previous commander had certified that we had 100 percent accountability of our agent stocks. The disconnect? When the institute conducted the prior inventory, it started with the list and compared it with the vials, not the other way around. This was a self-inflicted wound.

The army previously required an SIR for any "underage" (i.e., missing vials), which made sense, because a vial could have been stolen. But just days before, as part of the new post-Ivins rules, it had decided to do one better than all other research labs and *added* a new rule, requiring an SIR for any "overage" (i.e., extra vials found that were not in the database).[5]

The army had painted us into a corner. I knew immediately that we had no choice but to shut down the entire institute and conduct a full inventory. The four vials called into question our entire inventory database.

After a brief discussion of an action plan but feeling the weight of the news we would bring him, the three of us slumped silently, like condemned prisoners, over to the commander's office. He took the information in stride and agreed on the only path forward: shut down operations and conduct the inventory.

How did we get there? Had we just been blowing off the regulations?

Prior to 2001 USAMRIID did not have an institute-wide database with a line-by-line inventory. There were no such requirements. Instead, investigators kept spreadsheets of their agents in the freezers and tracked their daily work in their laboratory notebooks as "working stock." However, after 2001 the institute made a concerted effort to develop an institute-wide inventory database.[6] During the transition from paper records to an electronic database in 2005, all vials may not have been entered because it was built with data from active researchers, not samples in deep storage no longer used, but whenever an unaccounted vial was found, the scientist entered it into the database.[7]

As one scientist noted angrily, "You had a situation at USAMRIID where you had decades of stuff in freezers that had never been formally inventoried, because business was not done that way back in the day—and then all of a sudden some bureaucrat bean counters try to implement some new unproven inventory system in a really short period of time. It was destined to fail from the start."

Shutting down for the inventory would bring our $125 million research mission to a standstill. We braced for the backlash from unhappy research funders, the army's chain of command, and disgruntled scientists, who viewed the shut down as punishment.

Dave fired off another SIR up the chain, and that afternoon the commander emailed the institute explaining the situation: The institute must certify "that the full contents of each freezer and refrigerator have been evaluated and that all BSAT [Biological Select Agents and Toxins] are included in our inventory."[8]

Unfortunately, he didn't anticipate that one of our own would forward his email to the press. Once again we found ourselves in the media spotlight, gracing the front pages of the *Washington Post*, which painted a big target on us.

It might seem simple on the surface, but this would be a massive operation—to assess nearly six hundred freezers and fridges institute-wide, with over two hundred in the containment labs.

The commander tasked me to get the ball rolling. In some ways this would be my final leadership "exam."

During my years at USAMRIID, I had worked to protect the soldiers, the lab workers, the president, and ultimately, the nation. We had even managed to weather the Bruce Ivins anthrax crisis. Now I felt the weight of the institute's future on my shoulders. We had to get this right for USAMRIID to survive.

So, where to begin? I knew I needed someone to take my guidance and to "run point" for me who could interface with the lab scientists every day.

Colonel Terry Besch was a veterinarian with wide-ranging experience who had worked in the containment labs. She had impressed me with her insightful comments at meetings and by her candor in private. Tall, with short chestnut-colored hair, she had the right no-nonsense attitude. Although she ran a large support division for the institute, she had some good leaders working for her, so I thought she had some flexibility. I brought Terry into my office and asked her to run this to ground. Surprisingly, she seemed enthusiastic to take it on.

I wanted every freezer and refrigerator in the institute emptied and all contents moved into an empty freezer or fridge—on the hot side, gray side, and cold side (i.e., no "stone" would be left unturned). We needed a standardized, defensible process, and I didn't want to ever have to repeat this. We also needed to protect the commander, whom the army could punish as the fall guy at any time.

We developed the inventory process from scratch, with a strong sense of urgency and common sense. BSL-3 procedures came first, followed by BSL-4, then BSL-2. Before beginning we assessed what research absolutely could not be shut down, due to significant costs or if animals had already been infected with an agent. We did not want to harm animals unnecessarily. We emphasized accuracy over speed, but we couldn't risk having the virus and bacteria samples thaw during the transfers, or we might lose valuable historical samples.

Picking Terry to head the effort and giving her the authority to make decisions turned out to be one of the best decisions I had ever made. Terry laid out a large institute floor plan on my conference table. She numbered and tracked the locations of all the refrigerators and freezers and organized them according to which division would oversee the inventory in a specific area. Terry color-coded a freezer map, which looked like a Christmas display, showing "Green (complete), Yellow (in progress), and Red (pending start)," for lab rooms across the institute.

It has been said that no battle plan ever survives first contact with the enemy.[9] Every laboratory had its own idiosyncrasies that had to be accommodated, so Terry and I met regularly to adjust as issues came up during the execution of our "battle plan."

Until we rolled up our sleeves, we had no idea how long it would take.

At the start, we were hampered by the lack of empty freezers, even though we always kept a couple on hand, ready to go. It takes several hours to bring a freezer down to the proper temperature of minus eighty degrees Celsius, and just moving an eight-hundred-pound freezer into containment is a challenge that could take an hour or longer. After moving one into an airlock, the individual then changes and enters the lab, pulls the freezer in from the airlock, and searches for an available electrical outlet.

I placed an urgent priority 8 (critical) order with the contracting officer for twelve more freezers. She put in the order that day, but the government contract rules for mandatory competition kicked in. We waited . . . and waited. The freezers arrived over six weeks later. By then we had improvised without them.

Terry made a rule that every freezer had to be thawed and cleared with a squeegee to verify that every drawer was empty. Most researchers didn't like that. One researcher was particularly vocal, until one day, while using a squeegee in BSL-4, a vial popped out and hit the visor of her space suit. After that the complaints stopped.

Investigators are natural pack rats. The process was like cleaning out the attic. There was no telling what treasures we might find. During the inventory we "rediscovered" one set of valuable serum samples from Korean War veterans who had been infected with Korean hemorrhagic fever in the 1950s. Such samples, if destroyed, could never be replaced. The challenge is predicting which ones will be needed for future outbreaks or research.

The commander received constant pressure from up the chain of command: *When will this end?* He avoided making promises, but the pressure mounted. Terry and I authorized research operations in the containment suites to resume on a rolling basis as soon as we completed and validated each inventory.

One of Terry's update reports noted, "The amount of paperwork generated is extraordinary. Morale is low. People are frustrated." As the weeks went by, Terry's map showed the sea of red slowly transition to yellow, then green. Thankfully, the army surgeon general was our best supporter. I was occasionally copied on his messages to the vice chief of staff of the army, and I admired how quickly he understood our challenges and defended us. The USAMRIID commander extracted a huge concession during the inventory: if we noted any missing vials, we would send up an SIR immediately, but we could wait to report newly found inventoried vials in a single SIR at the end of the inventory. We could have been tied up in knots sending SIRs otherwise.

The commander's leaked email about the inventory forced us to engage with the media. The commander was under a lot of pressure, so Caree, our public affairs officer, asked me to serve as the media spokesperson instead. We had worked together previously on several interviews and press releases, so I knew she would keep me out of trouble, and she knew I wouldn't say anything stupid.

I looked forward to telling our side of the story and explaining its enormous challenges. I also believed that by serving as the spokesperson, I might take the "fall" if the army needed a scapegoat, rather than the commander.

Caree, Dave Shoemaker, and I sat around my conference table for a phone interview with a reporter from *Science* magazine. I took the "hot seat" and did most of the talking. The interview went well, and the reporter gave us a fair shake in his article for identifying a problem and addressing it, noting, "Researchers affected by the new rules are understandably unhappy, says Kortepeter, but they 'realize the importance' of carrying out the inventory."[10]

Four months after we began the inventory, we had counted and recorded over 70,000 vials and tissue samples of infectious pathogens. Among these, 9,220 vials had not previously been listed in the database. There were zero missing vials.

We weren't surprised to find some vials, but that number shocked even us. It is easy to ask, "how could this happen," but the changing rules added to the complexity—for example, genomic DNA for certain viruses was new on the inventory list, and many of the vials "found" were working stock. When a scientist pulled a vial out of the freezer, he or she could make additional samples from that vial and use those samples for experiments for up to thirty days before entering them in the database. It is easy to understand how a sample might be put back into the freezer and later forgotten without being entered into the database. The number of vials was constantly changing as a result.

The inventory was an incredible undertaking of time and resource allocation to complete, transfer all the agents between freezers, and update the computer catalog and agent storage after over forty years of collection. Terry tracked the effort, which required 223 people (~27 percent of the institute employees), and over 6,600 personnel hours at a cost of nearly $400,000, which was most likely an underestimate. The less tangible but larger opportunity cost was delaying our research mission by about one calendar quarter, which included damage to our credibility in the eyes of the country, the scientific community, the research funders, the army; disgruntled employees; and potential damage to critical frozen agent stocks.

As the inventory wound down, the media came calling again. We had to engage, but I worried that this time that things could get bloody.

Caree and I decided that I would lead the call again, but we pulled in a couple of others for backup. Once again we sat around my conference table: Caree, Terry Besch, Dave Shoemaker, and Sam Edwin, who was our lead on select agent inventories.[11] We spoke with reporters from the *Associated Press*, the *Frederick News Post*, the *Washington Post*, *Science*, and *Science Times*. As the call commenced, Dave later told me that he was thinking, *God, I'm glad it's Colonel Kortepeter, not me!* This time the USAMRIID commander sat on the periphery in my office during the discussion.

I emphasized that we had recognized a problem and addressed it head on. The news reports, however, didn't see it that way. The next day our 9,220-vial inventory discrepancy hit the major news outlets like a stink bomb. The sheer number of vials led to fresh scrutiny, and some reports made it sound as if we were trying to skirt the rules, which was not the case.[12]

The commander never said anything to me about how I handled the media call, but I wondered if I should write my own "I will get fired today" note in my daily notebook.

The inventory mismatch forced us to address something that should have been done several years earlier, but it also allowed us to catch the institute up with the new army rules. We were in a no-win situation, though, with strong disincentive previously to cease operations because the funding stream for USAMRIID had become tenuous, and if USAMRIID was not operational and couldn't do the work, funders would go elsewhere.[13]

The inventory results also reflected negatively on the CDC's laboratory inspection unit, the DSAT (Division of Select Agents and Toxins). As one article noted: "USAMRIID's case raises questions about lab inspections conducted by federal agencies to ensure compliance with select-agent rules. At least in USAMRIID's case, a CDC inspection in September 2008 failed to identify the problem of unlisted samples."[14]

Not surprisingly the CDC sent us a memo shortly thereafter, warning of another inspection. From that day on, the punishment continued. The CDC, as well as other agencies, including our parent command, the Department of the Army Inspector General's office, and others, have conducted nonstop inspections.

In the aftermath, the deputy to the army inspector general (DTIG), a two-star general from the Pentagon, visited us for a briefing on the situation. When an army unit does target practice, the DTIG noted, they check weapons out to the soldiers and issue bullets at the rifle range. At the end of the training, everything is returned and counted. The DTIG chastised us, saying that counting vials should be like counting bullets.

I disagreed, which probably didn't earn me any points with him or our chain of command, but he had a fundamental misunderstanding of the problem because he had never set foot inside a laboratory. "Bullets don't reproduce," I explained. Live agents do. Therefore, the focus on counting vials is misguided.

Under the right conditions, 2 bacteria dividing exponentially every twenty minutes could increase to over 65,000 in four hours. Viruses infect cells and produce millions of offspring. We can count all the vials we want, but a criminal who knows what he is doing doesn't have to steal a vial to produce thousands of vials of organisms. He or she only had to steal some ice crystals in the vial that contain organisms. The vial and the fluid level inside it would remain intact. Therefore, we should focus instead on what agents are used or stored in the lab and ensure that we have redundant measures to prevent the wrong people from getting near them.

In the meeting, one of my virology colleagues, Gene Olinger, displayed a diagram to illustrate an even bigger challenge for the DTIG. Like a New York City subway map, numerous colored lines crossed and spread out in all directions showing where numerous blood, tissue, or other body-fluid samples from infected animals went after a single experiment: to the diagnostics lab, pathology, the genomics lab, electron microscopy, and multiple refrigerators and freezers throughout the institute. Should every one of those pieces be counted, weighed, and tracked? Every scientist would need a full-time cadre following him or her around like a swarm of bees around honey, writing down everything the scientist was doing and entering it into a database. Such a protocol is not only very expensive, it is also dangerous because having more people in the containment lab just to gawk increases the safety risk for everyone. Under such circumstances it isn't long until research shuts down.

So in the long run, our rules risk shackling us, and we become less secure because we don't have the flexibility to respond quickly to a new outbreak, because we're so worried about watching our backs.

The DTIG was unmoved, saying, "I understand it's hard, but you need to find a way to do it."

I was proud that USAMRIID weathered the storm and resumed operations, but we had dodged a bullet. We witnessed what could have happened if we had failed: the army surgeon general shuttered the Armed Forces Institute of Pathology's (AFIP) decades-old biodefense program, and it had to transfer most of its pathogens to USAMRIID. The transfer of AFIP's samples demonstrated the army's renewed confidence in our ability to manage the inventory going forward.

The army and the navy also operate research institutes overseas in collaboration with foreign governments and militaries. One lab in Bangkok, Thailand, the Armed Forces Research Institute of Medical Sciences (AFRIMS), has served as a hub for infectious disease research throughout Asia for over fifty years. It faced the same challenges that we had dealing with select agents. When a team from the army inspector general paid the lab a visit, they found vials of *Bacillus anthracis* (anthrax) and *Yersinia pestis* (plague) bacteria and Crimean Congo hemorrhagic fever virus in the freezers. Their largest cache of select agents consisted of over three thousand Japanese encephalitis virus (JEV) isolates and animal tissue samples. Even though JEV is not usually considered a bioweapons threat, it had been classified as a select agent back in 2005.

JEV occurs throughout East Asia (Japan, China, Indonesia, India), generally in rural areas where pigs live close to humans, because pigs generate virus like a factory and the mosquitoes that spread the virus breed in the rice paddies nearby. JEV causes an infection of the brain leading to death or severe brain damage. Fortunately, not everyone who gets infected gets sick, and there is a vaccine to prevent it.

Colonel Fernando Guerena was an athletic Mexican American with black hair and a heavy accent who would later come to USAMRIID to take my old job as Medicine Division chief. Fernando was a veteran of the Iraq and Somalia operations and knew how to get things done. As the army officer put in charge of developing a program to handle the select agents at AFRIMS, he went about establishing the appropriate security and getting people enrolled in the PRP while the institute started to build a new BSL-3 containment laboratory. He told his personnel, "We can do this," noting, "It was a great exercise, because one day we'll have the real thing."

Despite Fernando's heroic efforts, when the new army requirements came out, overnight samples of JEV that had been stored inside AFRIMS freezers, probably for decades, were suddenly deemed unsafe. He recalls getting a memo on Cinco de Mayo from his commanding general directing AFRIMS to secure all the select agents immediately. A later memo directed him to destroy the samples. The staff searched the freezers and refrigerators and gathered all the samples of *B. anthracis*, *Y. pestis*, and Crimean Congo hemorrhagic fever virus that had been collected over decades, placed them in an auto-clave, and threw the switch that summarily destroyed them. Only the JEV samples would be spared.

Kurt Schaecher, another future USAMRIID colleague, was working at AFRIMS at the time on malaria countermeasures as the deputy chief of immunology and medicine. A man with short, graying hair and a robust sense of humor, he recalls getting the notification that AFRIMS needed to secure the JEV samples, package them up, and ship them out to USAMRIID. "We got caught with our pants down having it there," Kurt says. The notion that a terrorist would break into the lab and steal JEV samples that could be found easily in the local region seemed ridiculous. Nevertheless, the army officers saluted and did what they were told. The new army rules required someone to have "eyes on" the samples 24/7. Because the lab didn't have a video monitoring system, the institute consolidated all the JEV samples into two freezers in a room with glass doors. Kurt, Fernando, and their medical and scientific army colleagues had to keep guard on the samples 24/7. Kurt says, "I had to take a chair and sit in front of the room and just sit there." Fernando said it was like being on call. Some soldiers had the overnight shift and brought in their sleeping bags, teddy bears, and books during their guard shifts.

The lab was ordered to ship the JEV specimens from Thailand, a country where JEV already "lived" in nature, to USAMRIID in a country free of the disease (but harboring the mosquitoes that spread it), just to "check a box." When West Nile virus first landed in New York City in 1999, it took only a few years for mosquitoes to spread it across the entire country. If JEV got out, those same mosquitoes could sweep it across the country like a jetliner. It seemed foolish to risk a repeat of that with JEV. I objected. I lost the battle. Sometimes our rules get ahead of common sense.

When the Royal Thai Army Medical Department learned about the plan to ship the JEV specimens, it put the brakes on the operation, claiming ownership of the samples for Thailand, where they had been collected. Pathogen samples can have significant commercial value. The AFRIMS team kept the U.S. ambassador informed, but the two countries could not agree on ownership. They essentially agreed to disagree. Eventually, the Thai army allowed AFRIMS to move the samples temporarily to the United States, with the promise that they would be returned when the AFRIMS lab could meet all the new army rules.

Before shipping the samples, because of their presumed dangerous nature, a huge paperwork exercise ensued, including the need to complete endangered species importation paperwork because the samples included JEV-infected monkey tissues. Additionally, the samples had to fly using an airline "white glove" service that came with a special fee. Just getting the samples to the airport required armed guards. Each of the armed guards and anyone else who would transport the samples had to be drug tested, but there was no U.S. drug testing facility in Thailand. Fernando eventually managed to get them tested by none other than the antidoping agency from the Olympic committee stationed in Bangkok.

One evening Dave Shoemaker, my operations chief, brought me two sealed boxes, each about the size of a large sheet cake, containing the JEV samples that had arrived by courier from Thailand. I told him I didn't want anyone opening the boxes, let alone touching the samples inside. It was late in the day. Reminiscent of the final scene of *Indiana Jones* inside the vast warehouse full of stacked wooden crates, we carried those boxes down the institute's dark hallways to a lonely narrow side corridor behind a locked metal-mesh door. We unlocked one of the freezers and shoved the unopened boxes into an empty bottom drawer; then we locked it back up.

Years later they were shipped back to Thailand.

JEV would be removed from the select agents list three years later, in 2012.

I shudder to think how many irreplaceable historical specimens had to be destroyed, in haste, in the name of security. Which ones might be needed as a reference in future natural or bioterrorist outbreaks? We have no idea what samples our adversaries might be hiding in *their* freezers.

The military wasn't the only agency caught in the crossfire of new regulations. Years later I watched with empathy and understanding in 2014 as my colleagues at the NIH and the CDC also struggled with inventory and select agent issues. The NIH discovered twelve boxes with 327 vials holding a variety of pathogens, including small-pox and Q fever, a lesser-known potential bioweapon agent. This occurred around the same time that the CDC director had to testify before Congress about its mishandling of live anthrax and avian influenza samples.[15]

In August 2009 I concluded a tumultuous year as USAMRIID's deputy commander—a year where USAMRIID was shaken to its core by the Ivins and inventory challenges. I like to think I made a difference in helping to save this vital national resource from ruin.

During my next assignment, at the Uniformed Services University, the entire world would struggle with a new and unexpected disaster.

22

Behind the Scenes of Pandemic Response

Emile Ouamouno was probably no different from any other West African two-year-old, but shortly after coming down with fever, vomiting, and blood in his stool, he died on December 6, 2013, in Guinea, West Africa. Within days his pregnant mother, three-year-old sister, and grandmother also died. Although unrecognized at the time, Emile had spread Ebola virus infection to his family members and launched the largest outbreak of Ebola in history, larger than all previous Ebola outbreaks combined, with over twenty-eight thousand infected and over eleven thousand dead. Authorities would eventually label him "patient zero," the index case where it all began. How did he get infected? We don't know but suspect he had exposure to the virus near a tree infested with bat guano where he played.

Most prior outbreaks of Ebola occurred in remote African villages. As the hospital workers got infected and died, victims would avoid the hospitals. Eventually, without new, fresh victims, the outbreak burned itself out. Something different happened in West Africa, though. The environmental piece of the epidemiologic triangle (host-pathogen-environment) was primed for disaster. The health-care and public health systems had been decimated by years of civil war, so they were completely unprepared for Ebola. The outbreak started in Guinea, then moved to Liberia and eventually to Sierra Leone. A mobile population transited across the porous borders and from the jungle to the capitals and back, increasing the opportunity for fresh victims and ongoing spread of contagion. In some communities cultural burial practices that included very close contact with the dead body, which is teeming with Ebola virus, helped fuel the outbreak.

In the initial phases of illness, the infection doesn't spread efficiently, so if a patient is brought to the hospital early, close family members may be spared infection. But if they hide the victim at home, because they don't trust the government or believe community misinformation and rumors, they become the next victims as their family members pump out massive amounts of virus in diarrhea, vomit, or blood.

The outbreak was not recognized until mid-March 2014. By then it had been cooking for three to four months. Prior Ebola outbreaks had been managed largely by WHO, with Doctors without Borders (Médecins sans Frontières [MSF]) providing patient care, and in-country partners with the CDC chasing down potential patients in the community to quell the spread. By midsummer of 2014, the number of victims shot past one thousand. It was clear this outbreak wasn't going away. MSF and WHO, who usually minimize contact with the military, were overwhelmed and made unprecedented pleas for help from the U.S. and other militaries.

By this time I was serving as the associate dean for research at the Uniformed Services University's Medical School. I had also picked up two new duties as the army surgeon general's consultant for biodefense and as co-chair of the Biomedical Advisory Panel of the North Atlantic Treaty Organization (NATO), which kept me engaged with Ebola.

As we watched the West Africa outbreak unfold, my DoD medical colleagues and I welcomed the WHO invitation and were anxious to get to Africa to assist.

The DoD response planning kicked into high gear. I joined an endless stream of conference calls with Health and Human Services and State Department actors in addition to meetings with the Pentagon's DoD Ebola Working Group. Two other colleagues and I rotated sending weekly summaries to the army surgeon general and other senior DoD leaders.[1] In an early-August weekly update, the summary noted, "There is considerable enthusiasm among the Army ID provider ranks and across the services, to assist in Africa."

We were receiving a constantly evolving list of "asks" from other agencies for different-sized medical facilities—twenty-five-bed, one-hundred-bed, two-hundred-bed hospitals as well as mobile laboratories. Our military infectious disease community came together once again. After several meetings and phone calls among our key leaders, I drafted a consensus memo that offered three potential levels of clinical "packages" to senior military leaders to send some of us to Africa. I launched it up the chain of command in late August.[2]

The same three of us attending the DoD Ebola Working Group meetings were asked to put together slides for a briefing on Ebola for the army's chief of staff. Good news. Things were looking favorable for us going to Africa.

Sadly, somewhere along the way up the chain there was a disconnect. By the time the chief of staff's personnel made their edits, our slides were unrecognizable. None of us were invited to the briefing. I don't know what happened in the interagency shooting matches behind closed doors, but rather abruptly the Pentagon blocked our medical personnel from going to Africa to assist with patient care, opting to focus on logistical functions, building Ebola treatment units, and providing training on personal protective equipment instead.

On September 9, 2014, the *Washington Post* noted: "The United States is hamstrung by a lack of military medical personnel with expertise dealing with the deadly virus, a top official [from the U.S. Agency for International Development] in charge of coordinating the U.S. response said Tuesday: *There isn't an existing cadre of people who have experience in treating this epidemic* other than the aid group Doctors Without Borders."[3]

Really?

Clearly, this government official was misinformed, or it was a feeble attempt to justify a decision already made. Military docs have a strong track record of going where needed and completing the mission, especially in austere environments. Despite all the hype about Ebola, we know how it spreads in a hospital, so it is possible to contain it if you treat it with respect. After all, who knew Ebola better than USAMRIID, which had set the "gold" standard with decades of experience conducting research and preparation for Ebola patients since the Slammer opened in 1972? USAMRIID also had an Aeromedical Isolation Team fielded for years for medically evacuating Ebola patients.

The death knell for military physicians to assist in Africa came during one of our Ebola Working Group meetings in early September at the Pentagon. The meeting summary stated, "There will be no DoD medical planner asked for or welcomed."

It was an incredible missed opportunity for military physicians to help with the outbreak and gain valuable experience caring for victims. Only two military ID docs would get to assist with patient care on the ground through their connections with WHO before the window was closed.[4]

Over the course of the summer, considerable international debate raged about the ethics and challenges of using unlicensed products (especially those that had never been tested in humans) to treat or vaccinate patients in such an austere environment. But as the number of victims continued to climb, it was no longer a question of if but when those therapies would be used. If we didn't lean forward and offer reasonable alternatives, desperate locals were already reaching for any kind of snake oil they could get their hands on. My colleagues and I still hoped to help with a research mission to understand how to improve patient survival.

The DoD had spent millions of dollars to develop vaccines, diagnostics, and treatments for Ebola. It was an unprecedented opportunity to finally test the promising ones in humans. It made sense for military physicians and scientists to be involved. We started planning for possible research studies. I drew on my experience on the SMART-IND team in discussions with the CDC and NIH colleagues on how to conduct research in an austere environment.

Unfortunately, by cutting us out of patient care, the DoD also cut us out of the African clinical research mission. Nevertheless, USAMRIID provided critical assistance for training deploying medical providers from other agencies on personal protective equipment, and army and navy lab teams launched to West Africa to provide badly needed diagnostics for patients in-country.

At the request of the ambassador, USAMRIID science colleagues Lieutenant Colonel Kurt Schaecher and Dr. Randy Schoepp, along with former USAMRIID colleague Dr. Lisa Hensley (now at the NIH), brought their expertise to Liberia in mid-2014 to perform Ebola lab diagnostics for patients. Ironically, Randy had operated out of a field site in Sierra Leone for years. He had published a research study from blood collections years before showing that some West Africans had antibodies to Ebola.[5] His results were greeted initially with skepticism by some. No longer.

Kurt Schaecher describes his experience with the lab in Liberia: "They needed help at the lab desperately, and they weren't able to keep up with the testing. They were running out of reagents, and they needed extra training." Before the team arrived, it was taking a week for the doctors to get diagnostic reports back from the lab about who was positive or negative for Ebola. By then it was too late, as many of the patients had already died.

Kurt noted a horrific scene when he entered the Liberian lab where his team planned to set up shop. The only working bathroom had stacks of open coolers for transporting patient samples covered in blood. The team put on protective equipment, decontaminated the coolers, and put them back in a safer, contained part of the lab.

Initially the lab received just a couple of samples a day, but that quickly escalated exponentially until they were getting dozens of samples daily for testing—*all positive* for Ebola. Samples would arrive wrapped in bandages or with patients' names written by hand on pieces of paper cut from old posters. The team visited the main hospital to assess how patient blood draws were being managed. They met Dr. Kent Brantley there, who was already ill at the time but didn't know he had Ebola.[6] Kurt showed me a picture of himself and Randy Schoepp—neither wearing personal protective equipment— just inches away from Dr. Brantley.

Kurt recalls getting Brantley's blood—marked with a different name, for privacy purposes. The first day it was negative. The next day, positive. Dr. Brantley would be the first Ebola victim medically evacuated back to the United States, in addition to receiving the first doses of a new monoclonal antibody "miracle drug," ZMapp.[7]

The lab, like everywhere else in Liberia, was powered only by a generator. The lab team had no armed guards to protect them—only a Liberian man with a club. Kurt told his colleagues that if they saw the guard screaming and running, they needed to run, too. They had found a trail that ran from the lab about a kilometer down the road to an old UN station manned by Nigerian soldiers. That was their destination if they had to evacuate quickly.

With my experience working with USAMRIID's Slammer, I was among a small cadre in the United States and Europe who believed in the concept of "biocontainment"—that it is advisable to care for Ebola victims in hospital isolation units specially designed to reduce the risk of spread to the healthcare providers.

Before Dr. Brantley was medically evacuated to the United States, I received a call one night from a reporter, because he had read my article describing how we managed the Slammer admission years earlier. He wanted to verify the existence of specialized biocontainment patient units in the United States. Like a good soldier, I asked permission from DoD public affairs before responding. My simple request went all the way to the Pentagon. I was told I could only confirm "on background" their existence, meaning the reporter couldn't use my name. Two days later he called back and wanted to interview me for a more detailed article. This time, public affairs responded that the CDC had the lead, and it wanted to ensure that the government spoke with "one voice." *Hmm*, I thought. I was beginning to wonder if we were even a part of that "voice."

The Slammer's capabilities were based on the BSL-4 biocontainment laboratory.[8] The CDC's original infection-control recommendations from the early 1980s for Ebola and other viral hemorrhagic fevers followed this model and recommended care in a "Vickers" unit. Like something out of *The Andromeda Strain*, a Vickers unit is a plastic chamber about the size of a coat closet that maintains a vacuum to the surrounding environment. Caregivers use plastic sleeves embedded in the chamber's envelope to care for a patient, akin to working in a glove box. This method may work in a hospital, but it is impossible to replicate the Slammer or a Vickers unit in a remote setting during an outbreak. Other means were sought and focused on several key concepts. Caregivers wore a combination of barriers, including gowns, gloves, aprons, face shields, and breathing masks. They moved in isolation wards through clean (i.e., "cold") areas to contaminated ("hot") areas, and then they were decontaminated upon exit, usually with a bleach solution. These methods worked, by and large, but they could not eliminate health-care worker infections completely.

Consequently, our small cadre of biocontainment advocates believed that in a developed setting, like the United States, a more sophisticated hospital approach was needed, so the University of Nebraska, Emory University, and the NIH built their own special isolation units adapted from the Slammer model. Sadly, USAMRIID's Slammer was closed in 2011 for a combination of reasons, lack of funding and support from leadership, among others. I helped put a nail in the Slammer coffin. After managing Kelly's admission in 2004, when I returned as deputy commander in 2009, I had concerns that the Slammer was thirty miles from its parent hospital, Walter Reed Army Medical Center. Although everything worked out for Kelly's care, I believed that an isolation unit was more appropriately housed within a hospital rather than a research lab, and I feared that if Kelly had had a bad outcome, we would have been faulted. I briefed our commanding general about my concerns. At the end of my brief, he said, "I want to get out of the Slammer business."

Meanwhile, over four decades, the CDC's recommendations for infection control became more in line with the field model, rather than the Slammer model.

As the outbreak raged on, and the risk of Ebola patients coming to the United States increased, the CDC director echoed the less-rigorous field model when he testified before Congress that "any hospital can care for Ebola." When I heard that, I thought, *Oh, really?* That was a particularly concerning statement, especially given how efficiently Ebola can spread through an *unprepared* hospital ward. At the time the medical community in the United States was inexperienced with Ebola. I knew I had to take action.

Ebola is just too unforgiving. At the peak of infection, the convergence of millions of virus particles in a drop of blood, the few particles needed to infect, and victims expelling large amounts of body fluids (vomit, diarrhea) or bleeding create the perfect storm. There is no room for error. There is a reason that over five hundred health-care workers died from Ebola in the 2014–16 West Africa outbreak. This provided a warning about what we were dealing with.

After the Pentagon had blocked me from talking with the reporter previously, I realized I couldn't just pick up the phone to make an impact, but I wanted to sound the alarm and educate the medical community. So I enlisted colleagues at the University of Nebraska to join me in drafting an opinion piece for publication about the importance of specialized isolation units. We noted, "The serious nature of filoviral [Ebola, Marburg] and arenaviral [Lassa] infections, their rarity and unfamiliarity to clinicians in developed settings, the lack of effective treatments and vaccines, their propensity to infect health care staff, and the infection control challenges they present argue for, in our opinion, specialized containment and treatment facilities." In short, we meant, *Let the places that are familiar with this and train for it regularly handle it.*

I fired the article off to two top medical journals. Both rejected it. Undaunted, and recognizing the urgency, I launched it to the *Annals of Internal Medicine*, a highly respected journal. While it was being reviewed, Thomas Eric Duncan, a forty-five-year-old ill Liberian man, was admitted to Dallas Presbyterian Hospital. He had been seen in the emergency room several days earlier and sent home, despite mentioning his recent return from Liberia, one of the countries affected by the outbreak. My major concerns came to fruition when we learned that Duncan had infected two nurses with Ebola. The *Annals* recognized the significance of our article and published it online within hours—the fastest I've ever had an article published. The title of the article was "Caring for Patients with Ebola: A Challenge in Any Care Facility."[9]

The media picked up on our concerns, and one online piece headlined: "Top Federal Doctors Dispute CDC." The notion of containment care had a rebirth. After that, with one exception, all patients cared for in the United States were shipped to one of the three existing biocontainment units. One patient was cared for at Bellevue Medical Center in New York City, showing that other *prepared* facilities could do it right. In our article we also opined strategically about how to prepare for the next pandemic: "We envision the need for a network of strategically located regional referral centers serving designated catchment areas tied to BSL-4 laboratories or airport quarantine stations. . . . These could serve as national resources, coordinated through the Department of Health and Human Services and Centers for Disease Control and Prevention, with certification (much like trauma centers) to provide a higher level of care."

During the Ebola crisis, one afternoon while departing my son's Sunday afternoon baseball game, army colleague Stephen Thomas called my cell phone. He had received an email query from the army surgeon general because General Odierno, the army's chief of staff, wanted to know how we were going to protect the army communities when military service members building Ebola treatment units in Africa returned home. Stephen was weighing the pros and cons of whether the soldiers should be quarantined upon return. Drawing on my experience managing potential laboratory exposures at USAMRIID, I initially said that if the soldiers didn't interface with the population in Africa, their risk of exposure was extremely low. There would be no reason to quarantine them.

But as I considered this matter further, we had heard reports of military spouses who didn't want their soldier wives or husbands to come home for fear they would spread Ebola. Lassa fever was also endemic to West Africa. Victims don't need to have close contact with a patient to catch it—contact with rat urine or feces is sufficient, which posed a higher risk to our forces than Ebola. Moreover, we knew West Africa was a hotbed for malaria. We could not guarantee that the soldiers would take their malaria pills religiously, and we didn't want to repeat the "4M Disaster." I also worried that it would take only one soldier with Ebola to paint every soldier coming back with suspicion. Stephen also worried about multiple unknown risks of other infectious diseases and the potential for "mission creep." There was no telling what situations the soldiers might get into that could put them at risk. To make matters worse, significant chaos was at work in the United States as the civilian sector grappled with how to handle returning health-care workers. One nurse returning from West Africa who had no symptoms was forcibly quarantined by New Jersey governor Chris Christie after she landed in Newark.

As I added up these nuances, it became clearer to me that having soldiers remain under close observation ("quarantine") for two to three weeks upon return made sense. It would reassure the families that they had no risk. We could observe the soldiers for Lassa fever *and* Ebola, but even more importantly, also malaria. Stephen and I agreed. Once again the military infectious disease community came together and held a couple of conference calls and email exchanges to generate another consensus statement arguing for quarantine that went up the chain of command. Eventually it was dubbed euphemistically "controlled monitoring," but the army surgeon general and army chief of staff endorsed the idea. It became policy. Seven military bases with accessible hospitals were designated to handle the three-thousand-plus returning soldiers. The military took some heat from the medical and scientific community, but that blew over quickly because the policy worked like a charm. A survey of quarantined soldiers demonstrated general support for the policy: 72 percent thought it would "reduce anxiety in our communities," and a majority believed it would "keep our families safe." A surprising 20 percent thought it should be done for every deployment.[10]

The DoD played a significant supportive role that appeared to help turn the tide of the outbreak. The rapid diagnostic test that was used in the United States and Africa was developed by my colleagues at USAMRIID.

Although I was disappointed not to make it to West Africa for Ebola, I was glad that my knowledge and experience as well as the expertise of my colleagues helped to impact certain key aspects of the response back home. I was a member of a quick-response force for any DoD Ebola patients in the United States and participated in an international research team, led by the NIH, to assess whether the monoclonal antibody cocktail ZMapp worked for Ebola.[11] I also served as a consultant for my ID colleagues at Walter Reed National Military Medical Center as they reconfigured their ICU for possible Ebola patients.

•••

And there is a little-known story about Ebola, the army, and dogs . . .

Lieutenant Colonel Tony Alves, an army veterinary pathologist, is an athletic African American male who shaves his head and wears black-and-red running sweats when not sporting his military uniform. He has a rare skill set as a veterinary pathologist with BSL-4 laboratory experience. Although we have virtually eliminated the use of sharp objects in the containment laboratories, pathologists like Tony do some of the scariest things with scalpels. It's a job requirement. Consequently, they wear extra layers of purple nitrile gloves as well as a chain mail glove that looks like something the Knights of the Round Table might wear.

Tony's work in the BSL-4 lab makes him no stranger to Ebola—in fact he did some of the monkey necropsies for a study with me. So in the spring of 2014, as word spread about Ebola in West Africa, his ears perked up. By the time President Obama announced the deployment of thousands of troops into West Africa to build healthcare facilities, Tony had a particular concern. With his unique perspective as a veterinarian, army officer, and Ebola expert, he started to think about animals . . . dogs, in particular.

When the military sends special forces, civil affairs, or military police units overseas, a cadre of lesser-known, unique forces accompany them: military working dogs. These dogs hold a special status— they are not merely mascots—they have a bona fide mission and are treated as "comrades in arms," as important as any other soldier. I have personally witnessed the devastating effect on morale in a military unit when one of these "battle buddies" dies.

Tony started to think, "What is the risk to the dogs? Have dogs ever been sick with Ebola? Do they even get sick? If they don't get sick, could they still get infected, shed virus, and could they spread the disease?"

These were important questions. When he scanned the medical literature, he found only one study where a team of investigators drew blood on stray dogs in Gabon after an outbreak. Some of the dogs that had been foraging on human carcasses did have antibodies to the virus, meaning they had been infected, but there wasn't enough information to answer all of Tony's questions.

Concerned that military working dogs might accompany the U.S. forces to West Africa, Tony worried that we didn't understand their risk of infection, their risk of infecting the forces, or how to handle them when they returned to the United States. He asked the CDC if it had a policy on quarantine or testing pets with possible Ebola. It didn't, and it had no plans to develop one, because it was already knee-deep in human disease preparations.

Without any information to go on, Tony, who now worked in the army surgeon general's office, joined with his colleagues to draft an information paper. They recommended that until this issue could be sorted out, working dogs should not be sent to West Africa. This quieted things for the moment.

Then the bomb dropped. A nursing assistant in Spain got sick with Ebola. She recovered, but there was a catch. She had had contact with her pet dog at home. What should they do with the dog? Nobody knew. The Spanish authorities made the difficult decision quickly—they euthanized the dog, which caused a public outcry. It would be a disaster if that happened in the United States. Suddenly, the questions Tony had been asking needed answers.

Tony contacted his former colleague, Mark Wolcott, who ran the Special Pathogens Lab at USAMRIID. Mark and his colleagues had developed the Ebola test for humans. "Could you test [blood from a military working dog] to determine whether the Ebola test for humans would also work for dogs?" Tony asked.

Sure. No problem.

Tony hand-carried blood to USAMRIID from three military working dogs collected during the animals' routine exams. Inside the BSL-4 lab, the USAMRIID team "spiked" the blood with Ebola virus to come up with different concentrations of virus. Would the human PCR test pick up the Ebola?

Yes. It worked. The limits of detection in the dogs were similar to those in humans.

So far so good. Then the second bomb dropped. Thomas Eric Duncan, the severely ill man from Liberia was admitted to a hospital in Dallas, Texas, and died on October 8, 2014. He had infected two of the nurses caring for him with Ebola. On October 11 authorities realized that one of those nurses, Nina Pham, had contact with her pet dog while she had Ebola. Oh, shit! What should they do with the dog? The dog was moved to a quarantine facility in an old airfield in Texas. Soldiers guarding the dog wore full personal protective equipment and positive purified air respirators (PAPRs) as if the dog had Ebola.

On October 15 Tony's phone "blew up" with calls from the CDC. Could the army test blood, urine, and feces from Nina Pham's dog for Ebola? Just because a test works on blood doesn't mean it's going to work with other body fluids. The USAMRIID team was already one step ahead. They had previously obtained urine and feces from one of their lab technician's pet dogs and spiked those with Ebola to ensure that the test worked for those specimens as well as for blood. It did. All was good.

After several calls to coordinate shipping, blood, urine, and feces from Nina's dog arrived at USAMRIID for testing from the tenth and eighteenth days after the dog had been exposed to Nina. All were negative! The dog was Ebola free. The Texas authorities could then release the dog from quarantine. Pictures of Nina Pham smiling with her dog splashed across on the internet. It was a great interagency effort, with the USAMRIID team, Tony Alves and Mark Wolcott, as the heroes behind the scenes.[12]

In the aftermath Tony and colleagues from the army, USAMRIID, the CDC, and other agencies put together guidance for dog and cat quarantine after potential exposure to a human with Ebola. USAMRIID transferred their procedures to the CDC, so it could serve as the central referral point for anyone needing to test his or her pet. Problem solved.

The massive Ebola outbreak in West Africa is, thankfully, behind us. Unfortunately, we didn't use this unprecedented outbreak to full advantage. We learned that providing intensive care can significantly reduce the death rate. Even in the field, basic procedures such as measuring and correcting electrolyte imbalances in the blood can be beneficial. It was nice to see that the data from our monkey study years earlier, which suggested the benefit of IV fluids, was validated in humans. Sadly, we still don't have a magic bullet. One vaccine appeared to prevent spread of the virus to those exposed, and a monoclonal antibody cocktail looked promising, but its effectiveness wasn't proven. Many of the treatments we hoped would be beneficial ended up being anything but. Some of us have gone back to the drawing board to rethink approaches.

The work will continue, but we can't forget some of the key issues. Infectious diseases have no boundaries, so what affects people an ocean away can still affect us. Leadership and cooperation among multiple agencies can effectively shut down or limit the size of future outbreaks.[13] During subsequent Ebola outbreaks after the West Africa outbreak, WHO has taken a more aggressive approach earlier and incorporated research as a critical part of its responses. This is a good thing.

But what is the next threat? That is the million-dollar question.

23

Looking Forward—the Challenges Continue

Since I arrived at USAMRIID back in 1998, the threats we face from biological weapons have not significantly diminished. In fact they may have increased. Despite the recent discussions between the Trump administration and North Korea, a report by Harvard's Belfer Center released in October 2017 sounded the alarm about North Korea's potential biological weapons activities. Utilizing unclassified reports, defector testimonies, and interviews with subject-matter experts, the report authors argue that preparation for the biological weapons threat is "urgent and necessary."[1] Although the media has focused on North Korea's nuclear program, use of the nerve agent vx to assassinate Kim Jong-Un's half-brother in early 2018 should provide a wake-up call that we ignore North Korea's interest in other weapons of mass destruction at our peril.

Prior reports have noted North Korea's possession of and capability to cultivate thirteen agents, including some of the Chessmen on the category A threat list: Bishop Plague (*Yersinia pestis*), Queen Anthrax (*Bacillus anthracis*), King Smallpox (*Variola major*), and Pawn Botulism (*Clostridium botulinum*).

Possession is only one aspect. Weaponization and stabilization for deployment are others. The Belfer report notes that North Korea may have the capability to weaponize the agents. Deployment methods such as by rocket launchers, sprayers, or infected humans used as vectors are theoretical possibilities. The South Korean Ministry of Defense stated that the thirteen agents could be weaponized "within ten days."

The late William Patrick, chief of product development for the

United States' former offensive biological weapons program once told me that the U.S. program proved the effectiveness of biological weapons "beyond the shadow of a doubt." We don't need to experience a nightmare scenario on the Korean peninsula to prove Bill's point. As the Harvard report points out, we should not feel reassured just because we have limited intelligence on North Korea's capabilities. We should be even more concerned. Despite having suspicions about the former Soviet bioweapons program, we were still shocked at the extensive Soviet biological weapons arsenal revealed by Dr. Ken Alibek in his book *Biohazard*, after his defection in the 1990s.[2]

We don't have to look far to know that interest in deploying weapons of mass destruction is alive and well, with periodic chemical agent attacks occurring in Syria against civilian populations and the assassination attempt in 2018 on a former Russian spy in the United Kingdom with a Novichok nerve agent. We still don't have a window inside Russia's military bioweapons capabilities.

Even if we don't get hit with a bioweapon attack, we should have learned from Ebola, Zika, Middle East respiratory syndrome (MERS), and severe acute respiratory syndrome (SARS) that Mother Nature is a very efficient bioterrorist.

Clearly, the need for expertise and preparedness for emerging infectious diseases and bioterrorism has not diminished. We suffer the curse of always "preparing for the last war," and we do a poor job of predicting how, when, or where the next pandemic will start. It is merely a matter of time until the next mysterious illness emerges, leaving a trail of victims with symptoms that puzzle experts and terrify the public. We know only one thing for certain: something else *will* come along when we least expect it, and it will be something we don't anticipate.

The anthrax attacks and the Ebola outbreak in West Africa helped to kick-start improved infrastructure, disease surveillance systems, coordination, and technology for more rapid diagnostics and microbial forensics, but politicians have short memories, so knowledge of the threat doesn't necessarily translate to sustained funding for preparedness. At the same time, each new technology for improving diagnosis or scientific analysis brings a potential downside. The ability to manipulate genes has gotten easier with new genetic-engineering technologies such as CRISPR, making manipulation of harmful microbes accessible to a wider range of potential terrorists. The tools of microbiology also grow ever faster, smaller, and cheaper, so the notion of the bioterrorist making a weapon in his or her garage becomes more feasible every day.

We have some good news related to Ebola: a promising vaccine currently in use for the outbreak in the Democratic Republic of the Congo, as well as a couple of promising treatments. Early work for them was conducted at USAMRIID. We have a better system in place now to take orphan products past the difficult funding hurdles and human studies needed to get them licensed with the help of the Biomedical Advanced Research and Development Authority (BARDA), but at the same time, developing new vaccines and treatments remains difficult and very expensive. The terrorists have the advantage of selecting the agent they prefer, deploying it where we are most vulnerable, and not having to worry about regulations. And while we recognize better the importance of conducting research in real time during an outbreak to move products closer to licensure, it remains a formidable task to overcome cultural barriers, ethical challenges, and regulatory and financial hurdles rapidly enough to make a difference, especially in remote regions of the world, where unusual diseases surface frequently. And research will, appropriately, always take a back seat in priority behind caring for the victims and stopping the outbreak.

The challenges I describe in this book continue today. In order to continue developing bioweapon countermeasures, with each move made by the terrorists, our scientists need the flexibility to innovate in their countermoves, just like on a chessboard. This is as true for the military (perhaps more so) as it is for the civilian sector. Fear, rather than common sense, has created a suffocating regulatory environment around select agent use, to the point that it can leave our nation more vulnerable in the long run. We can't let fear of mistakes drive science and drive policy. Just transferring a single test tube of blood from an Ebola victim requires an eighteen-wheeler at a cost of $5,000–$15,000. "Zero tolerance" for laboratory errors is not good policy. People are fallible, so we must accept a measure of risk to get reward. We can't have a laboratory "stand down" for every potential lab exposure. That's like saying, "If you don't want to get hit by a car, then never leave the house." Scientists working in the laboratory interpret the message of punishment, so reporting mishaps goes underground and ultimately puts the laboratory researchers and everyone else at greater risk. When we work with deadly diseases, we shouldn't be surprised that some unexpected outcomes occur. The best policy is to learn from each error and design ways to mitigate future errors. Overall, we must remain vigilant and keep up the fight, lest the microbes and our adversaries win. In 2018 the White House released a new "National Biodefense Strategy" for a coordinated effort to accomplish the vision that "the United States actively and effectively prevents, prepares for, responds to, recovers from, and mitigates risk from natural, accidental, or deliberate biological threats." This is a step in the right direction, but we must remain mindful of the need to stop infectious diseases where they occur before they spread because they don't respect national or continental borders.

In 2009 Wendy Sammons-Jackson, an army major and microbiologist, was in her second tour of duty at USAMRIID. A medium-height runner, with bobbed blond hair and a perpetual smile, Wendy was enthusiastic about her first research project studying *Francisella tularensis* bacteria that might eventually lead to an improved tularemia vaccine. Wendy worked under the hood growing the *Francisella* organism in a broth culture and then carefully removing the fluid broth with a syringe and passing it through a filter. Before starting work, she was evaluated for possible vaccination against tularemia, but her blood tests showed she already had antibodies, possibly from a tularemia infection years prior, so she was not vaccinated.

On a Friday afternoon a week before Thanksgiving, Wendy began to feel ill, and her smile disappeared. It started with a headache, influenza-like symptoms, and diarrhea. Over the next two days, the headache worsened, like someone was beating her over the head with a hammer, and she had wide temperature swings three to four times a day, with fevers as high as 105 degrees. Loss of appetite and extreme muscle and joint pain in her ankles and hips knocked her flat, and she couldn't get out of bed.

She suffered at home through the weekend, and like a good soldier, she called in sick the following Monday and went to the clinic on Tuesday. It was the height of the 2009 swine flu epidemic. The doctor who saw her, understandably, presumed she had the flu. No lab tests were done, and she was sent home with the usual instructions to take ibuprofen as needed.

Thanksgiving approached, but because she felt too ill, she abandoned plans to host the family. Her mother volunteered to host in Delaware instead. Still ill with fevers and chills, Wendy managed to make the trip with her husband and two infant boys, even as she feared spreading the flu to other family members. While in Delaware she noticed new sharp pains in her chest when inhaling, which prompted a trip to a local emergency room. She explained to the doctor that she had been told she had the flu, but she now feared she might be developing pneumonia. The doctor took a chest X-ray, which was negative.

"Continue treating as you have been," he told her.

From there things went further downhill. The week after Thanksgiving, she couldn't catch her breath when she sat up. She called into work again—this time talking to one of USAMRIID's physicians. He expressed concern that her illness might not be the flu, but it could be related to her lab work. He told her to go to the hospital and that he and the other USAMRIID physicians would be standing by to talk to whomever she saw.

After she told the doctor in the internal medicine clinic about the pain, the fevers, and her fear of pneumonia, he told her that she didn't have pneumonia. Continue as you have. She pushed back, saying the USAMRIID doctors wanted to talk to him.

He was not interested. "I think you are stressed out taking care of your family and that's why you're not recovering."

Wendy pleaded with him to rule out tularemia. He said that she didn't even have a fever. She knew that, because the fevers were cyclical, but she assured him that the fever would return within the hour.

"Sometimes people think they have a fever when they have a hot flash," the doctor explained. He gave her a card and recommended stress-management counseling.

Desperate, Wendy called back to USAMRIID and the doctors

there told her to come to the institute immediately and had her get a chest X-ray at the neighboring clinic on Fort Detrick. The X-ray showed fluid and lymph node swelling inside her chest, along with pneumonia. After seeing this, USAMRIID docs started her on antibiotics and drew blood to test for tularemia. A couple of days later, the tularemia test came back positive. Her fever initially dropped on the antibiotics, but within days, she was feeling worse again, so she was finally admitted to the hospital. Her original chest X-ray was reevaluated and found to indicate pneumonia, which the emergency room staff had not picked up on. After several weeks of treatment and disabling side effects, Wendy gradually improved, but her odyssey would continue for another two years with low blood counts, ongoing fatigue, and pains in her back and joints.

Wendy's story is not that unusual. She considers that she might have had an earlier diagnosis if someone had actually tested her for influenza. A negative test might have prompted a search for an alternate cause, because once she had been labeled as having "influenza," it was hard for physicians to think otherwise. It wasn't until USAMRIID's physicians became involved that the course began to change. She also admits that, although she worried about the possibility that her illness could have been tularemia, she didn't want to believe that something she had done in the lab might have led to the exposure. The safety review never determined exactly how she was exposed, but a large instrument inside the hood at the time may have altered the normally protective air curtain. It was a small perturbation, but with an agent like tularemia, which only requires a few organisms to infect, it could make all the difference.

What if Wendy had shown up at a clinic with tularemia as a sentinel case after a bioweapon attack rather than from a laboratory-acquired infection? Would her illness have been recognized in time to prevent other illnesses? I like to think so, but I am skeptical. Just as in our phone call with Tom Brokaw back in 2001, it is hard to tease apart the important clues that might indicate we are dealing with the rare "zebra" instead of a more common ailment—hence the need to maintain an index of suspicion for the unusual.

Figuring out whether an outbreak is natural or spread by the enemy requires recognizing "red flags" that the outbreak was man-made. After an air attack, victims' locations at the time of the attack could show an illness pattern along a downwind plume. A higher death rate than usual could indicate that a pathogen has been manipulated to make it deadlier. A pathogen in a place it doesn't belong or multiple unexplained outbreaks should also ring alarm bells.

Many of the potential bioweapon threats, like anthrax, plague, and tularemia, preferentially infect animals over humans. So animal disease after or at the same time as infections in humans could be a clue of an intentional release. Of course the perpetrators make our job easier if they leave behind direct evidence, like the tainted anthrax letters or Dianne Thompson's pastries.

Determining scientifically that a bioweapon attack has occurred is not easy.[3] My colleagues and I tested a scoring method against six suspicious outbreaks.[4] Only the anthrax letter outbreak would have been categorized as "highly likely" due to bioterrorism.

So what is the solution?

Recognizing something unusual relies on a human putting two and two together. In 1994, while working in Florida, Dr. Scott Folk, an infectious disease doctor, treated a couple of patients severely ill with fevers, chills, headaches, muscle aches, nausea, low platelets, and liver injury.[5] They fit the pattern of a rickettsial illness, like Rocky Mountain spotted fever. The tests for such diseases came back negative, but the patients improved after he treated them with doxycycline, the antibiotic that usually works for rickettsiae. Puzzled, Dr. Folk contacted the CDC and they ran a battery of tests. They eventually made the diagnosis of a different rickettsial disease called Ehrlichia. Although Dr. Folk was not the first to discover the pathogen, it was new to his location, so he and his CDC collaborators published a couple of articles on it.

Fast forward ten years to 2004. Dr. Folk was then working in Missouri. Again, he saw a few patients with rickettsia-like symptoms, but something was amiss. They didn't respond to doxycycline as they had before, so he contacted his former CDC collaborators. This time, they grew a brand-new virus in the lab. They named it Heartland virus. Antibiotics don't work against viruses, so it was not surprising, in retrospect, that the patients didn't respond to doxycycline.

Dr. Folk's ability to make that discovery depended on a rare convergence of events: his experience *ten years* earlier, which primed him to consider something unusual, plus his access to sophisticated diagnostic testing through his preestablished contacts at the CDC. We need a similar convergence of events and experience to identify bioterrorist attacks early.

Surveillance systems are important for giving us normal disease rates in a specific population, so we have something to compare with before we sound the alarm. There is a tradeoff, though. The more sensitive we make a surveillance system, the more times we chase down false alarms. The less sensitive it is, the more we risk missing the outbreak early enough to make a difference. Surveillance systems, though, won't usually give us the early warning we need. Humans do that.

As two physicians noted in an article after the anthrax letter attacks: "Despite our significant advances in technology and the development of systems designed for bioterrorism preparedness, we firmly believe that an astute clinician will once again be the first to recognize the next patient with an illness resulting from deliberate exposure to a biologic agent. It has been said that luck is where the road of opportunity crosses the road of preparation. In public health this intersection is often at the bedside."[6]

I agree.

But it is more than luck. The physician at the bedside needs a trained eye to recognize the zebra, coupled with the determination to pick up the phone and call for help.

Afterword

....

Despite some of the challenges I have described, USAMRIID remains a critical national asset with amazing scientists and capabilities. USAMRIID continues as a leader developing countermeasures against Ebola and anthrax as well as many other diseases, like tularemia, encephalitis viruses, botulism, ricin, and plague. Work conducted at USAMRIID over decades has built a foundation for countermeasures for many of those diseases. Decades of Ebola studies there on the pathogenesis, pathology, pathophysiology, diagnostics, vaccines, and therapeutics are the reason we had any potential countermeasures to choose from during the 2014–16 West Africa Ebola outbreak. The vital work needs to continue.

If you were to visit Fort Detrick today, you would notice right behind USAMRIID a massive five-story building under construction, the "New" USAMRIID. When it is completed, it will contain the largest BSL-4 lab in the world. It is a hopeful sign, but USAMRIID doesn't often get the credit it deserves and the army does a poor job of recognizing and championing its "crown jewel" biodefense research facility a stone's throw from the Washington DC Beltway. This is unfortunate because with recognition comes resources. As Caree Vander Linden told me recently, "We always got beat up for doing the right things," but somehow we survived. "We're a resilient organization." That's a testimony to the people who have lived and worked there.

As the "old guard" who worked with me transition to retirement or transfer to one of the other containment labs around the country, the biggest challenges may be filling the institute with qualified scientists and paying the massive electricity bill.

A full list of USAMRIID's contributions to biodefense and science, in general, probably deserves its own book, but USAMRIID has had an incredible safety record for over forty-five years, despite countless employees working on extremely hazardous pathogens. It has also set the standard for things like containment care and aeromedical isolation for patients with highly hazardous communicable pathogens, which have now been replicated elsewhere. Probably its most important asset is the people who have worked there over the decades. They have made significant impact with their work at USAMRIID and also after moving to other containment laboratories across the nation at the NIAID, the CDC, and the University of Texas; to academia; and to the pharmaceutical industry. USAMRIID personnel have shared their expertise in containment lab safety and bioweapon inspections, produced educational materials on biowarfare and bioterrorism, provided diagnostic support for outbreaks, and developed vaccine protocols and products for outbreak response.

Whenever a new infectious disease crisis occurs, USAMRIID answers the call from the nation and the world, sometimes in the lead, sometimes in a supportive role. My hope is that USAMRIID remains the cornerstone for biodefense that will serve us well into the future, but it will take ongoing nourishment and support from the army. When the next emerging infectious disease or bioterrorism crisis occurs, the nation should continue to expect USAMRIID investigators to remain the nation's "Biohazard 911"—a response hotline, willing to drop everything to respond again to the nation's needs.

As for me, I joined the army in 1985 inspired to become Hawkeye Pierce from *M*A*S*H*, but as I left in 2016, my friends more rightly compared me with the Dustin Hoffman character from the movie *Outbreak*. Physicians in the army are taught that they are soldiers and officers first and physicians second. When I was a new division chief at USAMRIID, one of our commanding generals recited "I Am a Soldier" at a retreat with all his subordinate commanders. When the subordinate commanders took the stage, each began his or her remarks with the words "I am a soldier." It didn't resonate with me at the time; however, now that I am retired from the army, as I look back on my career, I realize how important it has been for me, and how proud I am, to be a soldier. It is truly in my blood.

I arrived at USAMRIID as a junior physician-officer wanting to do something important. My experiences reached far beyond my expectations, and I am grateful that my bosses, commanders, and generals along the way had the confidence to give me opportunities to lead, which gave me a seat at the table for some of the most exciting infectious-disease challenges of this generation. I left USAMRIID in 2009 with more gray hair and the scars of managing crises, but I wouldn't trade my experiences there. Some crises were real, others were false alarms, but we couldn't distinguish between the two as they began. Sometimes our preparations succeeded, other times not. But each time we came together, assessed the situation, and developed a response plan that worked.

I hope that my stories have given the reader a sense of the challenges and opportunities of working in this field and the numerous individuals who have dedicated their work and lives to this mission. I tried to give some of them a voice here, especially as they related to frustrations in the aftermath of the anthrax investigation. They are unsung government heroes dealing the best they can with difficult circumstances. The excitement I have had in my career was all about working with these friends and colleagues, our focus on the mission, and overcoming the shared challenges and frustrations together to make things better. Perhaps I am naive, but I hope that my stories inspire a new generation to work at one of the military's research labs or enter the fields of biodefense and infectious diseases. For me it has been quite an adventure.

I like to think I made a difference in the nation's preparedness for and response to biothreats and emerging infectious diseases. Although my career focused on those issues, at my core I am a physician who cares about people. Ultimately, I hope the beneficiaries of anything I have done are the patients—the soldiers, sailors, air force personnel, marines, and DoD civilians who willingly leave the protected confines of the outer perimeter in a hostile environment, trusting that we will use the best tools at hand to protect them and care for them when they become ill or are injured. We need to continue the scientific discoveries to protect them against the next biological weapon threat—and possibly against Mother Nature.

I spent my final tour in the military at "America's Medical School" at the Uniformed Services University of the Health Sciences (USU), where I ran an international infectious-disease research network and later became the associate dean for research. I transitioned out of the army in 2016, after twenty-seven-plus years, but I continue to collaborate with USAMRIID and USU colleagues, studying Ebola and training the next generation of military medical providers on biodefense. Through my current faculty position at the University of Nebraska's Medical Center and College of Public Health, where I work with a great group of colleagues at the National Ebola Training and Education Center (NETEC), I teach about infection control for disease outbreaks, conduct hospital preparedness consultations, and am helping to build a special pathogens research network. The vision we espoused in our article about biocontainment units has come to fruition. Through the work of the NETEC, the United States now has a hospital network with one designated biocontainment facility in each of ten emergency-response regions of the country. The focus of the network has expanded from Ebola to emerging infections. We don't know what the next infectious disease crisis will be, but it is guaranteed that it will be different from what we predict. Therefore, having a national platform for response and research is critical.

As I finish this book, a new Ebola outbreak that started in August 2018 is raging in the Democratic Republic of the Congo (DRC) with no end in sight. Sadly, despite having new tools (investigational vaccines and treatments) at our disposal, human nature continues to fuel the outbreak, which recently passed three thousand victims. Suspicion of the response teams on top of decades of civil strife have created the "perfect storm," where the responders and Ebola treatment units are being targeted directly in violent attacks, making this outbreak perhaps the most complex and challenging ever to control. I had the honor of leading Ebola infection control efforts for six weeks (December 2018–January 2019) for WHO in Burundi to prepare for a possible spillover from the neighboring DRC. This experience allowed me to make up for missing the chance to help out on the ground during the West Africa outbreak. Driving the mud-covered and pot-holed roads, visiting hospital wards, evaluating the Ebola treatment unit, and working with the local hospital, who, and ministry of health staff, I applied the different layers of skills that I had developed over decades for a very practical field mission. It was perhaps the most challenging and exhilarating work I have ever done.

Although I am technically "retired" from the military, my adventures continue. The work is too fascinating, and the opportunities, needs, and questions infinite, so it is hard to quit once you've caught the bug.

ACKNOWLEDGMENTS

I am thankful for my many colleagues and friends during my twenty-seven-plus-year army career who shared the daily challenges wherever we found ourselves, on the hospital wards or in the office, the lecture hall, the lab, cramped airplanes, dingy hotels, overseas training venues, a Humvee, a combat support hospital, a tent, or a bunker. I also thank my many mentors, supervisors, and commanders who gave me opportunities and put me in positions of responsibility that allowed me to grow as a physician, a soldier, an officer, and a leader.

I am grateful to the following friends and colleagues who took the time to share their memories with me, reviewed or corrected draft portions, or gave me supplemental documents that provided a more holistic and objective narrative: Arthur Anderson, Arthur Friedlander, Beverly Fogtman, Bret Purcell, Caree Vander Linden, Charles Hoke, David Shoemaker, Denise Clizbe, Derron (Tony) Alves, Dianne Negley, Ellen Boudreau, Fernando Guerena, Donald (Gray) Heppner, Greg Deye, Greg Martin, Henry (Hank) Heine, James Martin, Janice Rusnak, Jeff Adamovicz, John Aldis, John Grabenstein, Judith Pace-Templeton, Kelly Warfield, Kurt Schaecher, Pat Worsham, Phil Russell, Rich Trotta, Robert Kuschner, Scott Stanek, Stephen Thomas, Sybil Tasker, Terry Besch, Timothy Burgess, Tim Whitman, Tom Geisbert, and Wendy Sammons-Jackson. The following individuals reviewed the near-final full draft and gave me valuable feedback on how to improve it: Charles Hoke, Cynthia Williams, Ellen Boudreau, Erica Ragan, and Margie Dere. Charles and Ellen developed a standardized rating system that they applied to each chapter, which was incredible.

I would like to recognize my agent, Jim Hornfischer, a bestselling writer of naval war history, who saw potential in my initial email query and supported me to write the book I wanted to write. I also appreciate his introducing me to Kim Cross, author of the bestselling *What Stands in a Storm*. Kim helped me find my "voice" and served as my writing coach, and she encouraged me to interview others to improve the narrative with additional perspectives. She also shepherded me into the community of nonfiction writers and assisted me in crafting a solid book outline and proposal. Thanks also to Kim and my other colleagues at the Archer City Writing Workshop for taking me seriously, especially Glenn Stout, Brett Popplewell, and Wendy Reed, all talented writers and teachers, who provided critiques of my writing.

Thank you to Tom Swanson and the team at Potomac Books for taking a chance on an unknown writer with an interesting story to tell. Thanks especially to Abigail Stryker, who answered all my questions along the way, Barbara Wojhoski and Joeth Zucco for their skillful editing, and Jackson Adams and Tish Fobben for their marketing recommendations.

I would also like to thank the following people who assisted me with obtaining photos or photo permissions, although I may not have been able to use all the photos: Caree Vander Linden, who served as the facilitator for interviews with USAMRIID personnel and assisted with many USAMRIID photos, Barbara Richards, Charles Bailey, Charles Boles, Coleen Martinez, David Franz, David Tribble, Denise Clizbe, Donald (Gray) Heppner, Gene Olinger, John Dye, Kelly Warfield, Mark Takano, Pat Worsham, Rick Stevens, Robert Kuschner, Robert Rivard, Ted Cieslak, Tom Ksiazek, and Xiankun (Kevin) Zeng.

I appreciate the support and encouragement of many other friends, colleagues, and family members along the way who cheered me on when they heard I was writing this memoir.

Finally, I want to thank my wife, Cindy, who reviewed numerous manuscript versions and who took a chance on a lowly medical intern and left her family to live the army journey with me. She has tolerated the difficult role of the "trailing spouse" in the life of a soldier and physician with the late nights on call, middle-of-the-night emergencies, multiple moves, two deployments, and years of continuous travel, but she still managed to excel in her career, all while maintaining a solid home foundation for our three boys.

biological weapon or biological warfare (bw). A living pathogen or substance produced by a living pathogen (e.g., toxin) that has the potential to be used to cause illness or death in humans, animals, or plants. Certain characteristics may make a pathogen or toxin favorable for use as a weapon, such as stability, ability to disseminate by aerosol, high infection rate, person-to-person spread, ease of obtaining, and ability to grow in large quantities.

biosafety levels (bsl). Laboratory safety levels, ranging from 1 to 4. Pathogens are designated to be worked on under these levels, with the higher numbers reserved for more dangerous pathogens. Levels bsl-3 and bsl-4 are considered "containment" because pathogens at those levels cause potential risk by aerosol to laboratory workers.

category A threat agent. A list of six agents deemed by the cdc to have the potential to cause significant harm to a population. The diseases they cause are anthrax, botulism, plague, smallpox, tularemia, and viral hemorrhagic fever (Ebola, Marburg, Lassa). Also designated in this book as the "Six Chessmen."

chain of command. Higher levels within the military with authority over a specific military unit.

commander. The lead officer in a military unit who has disciplinary authority (under the Uniformed Code of Military Justice [ucmj]) over the personnel under his or her command.

deputy commander. The second in charge in a military unit. Can be designated as the acting commander, as needed. Often serves in the role of managing the daily operations of a military unit.

electrocardiogram (EKG). A method of measuring the electrical activity of the heart.

epidemiologic triangle. The three aspects needed to cause an outbreak: a susceptible host (human or animal), a pathogen, and the environment conducive to spread.

15–6 investigation. A formal military investigation into wrongdoing.

Food and Drug Administration (FDA). U.S. government agency that approves drugs, vaccines, and devices for use in the U.S. population.

hot side. The area in a containment lab where live, potentially deadly pathogens are worked with.

investigational new drug (IND). Designation given to vaccines or treatments that are not yet approved ("licensed") by the FDA. Any use of an IND in humans must be given under a protocol with appropriate informed consent of the volunteers receiving it.

Medical Research and Materiel Command (MRMC). Command organization one level up from USAMRIID. It is commanded by a two-star general.

quarantine. Restriction of movement and activities of a potentially infected individual who is not yet ill (originally on a ship for forty days) for a specified period of time to minimize risk of spread to others

select agent. A plant or animal pathogen deemed by the CDC and the USDA to pose a significant threat to human, animal, or plant health. These have special handling and transportation requirements.

Prologue

1. This term comes from Michael Crichton's book *The Andromeda Strain* (New York: Avon Books, 1969) about a deadly pathogen that comes to earth in a downed satellite.

2. Quarantine dates back to the Middle Ages period of the Black Death in Europe as a way to prevent the spread of illness. Ships would be required to retain their personnel on board for forty days to prevent the risk of bringing contagion on shore. It is used now to separate a person (who is not yet ill) who may have been exposed to a contagious disease from others for a specified period of time, depending on the particular disease.

3. Scott Stanek and I were division chiefs at the same time. Although the "Slammer" was physically located in the Medical Division clinic space when I was medical division chief, the Slammer space was under the control of Scott's Operational Medicine Division. Scott's division also had a cadre of enlisted soldiers and a nurse who were dedicated to an "Aeromedical Isolation Team" (AIT). The mission of the AIT was to travel anywhere in the world with a couple of hours' notice to pick up a potentially contagious casualty. Over the years they were put on alert several times for patients but were only activated for missions that did not involve a human patient (Operation Glove Box at Wright Patterson Air Force Base and for the Ebola virus outbreak in a nonhuman primate facility in Reston, Virginia, which was chronicled in Richard Preston's book *The Hot Zone*).

Even though Scott owned the Slammer space (and Jim Martin was the Slammer lead), the majority of the personnel who would be activated to assist during a patient admission worked for me as the Medicine Division chief. As such, given my role as the USAMRIID commander's senior medical advisor, the institute's clinical response fell under me.

4. Janice M. Rusnak et al., "Management Guidelines for Laboratory Exposures to Agents of Bioterrorism," *Journal of Occupational and Environmental Medicine* 46, no. 8 (2004): 801–11. See also Janice M. Rusnak et al., "Experience in the Medical Management of Potential Laboratory Exposures to Agents of Bioterrorism Based on Risk Assessment at the United States Army Medical Research Institute of Infectious Diseases (USAMRIID)," *Journal of Occupational and Environmental Medicine* 46, no. 8 (2004): 791–800.

5. The group included John Huggins, Tom Geisbert, George Ludwig, Alan Schmaljohn, Sina Bavari, Ellen Boudreau, Jim Martin, Scott Stanek, Mark Kortepeter, Jim Swearengen, and Ed Anderson.

6. This particular virus was slightly different from the "parent" Ebola Zaire virus. The virus was isolated from a human infected during the original 1976 Ebola outbreak in the Democratic Republic of Congo (previously Zaire). It was then "adapted" to infect mice in order to test potential countermeasures.

7. This scene is captured in David Quammen's book *Spillover* (New York: W. W. Norton, 2012), in which I am referred to as the head of the Medical Division: "The head of the Medical Division took Warfield into his office, sat her down, and gently told her the recommended next step. They wanted to put her in the Slammer" (106).

1. Beginnings

1. My former boss Kelly McKee was an experienced researcher on viral hemorrhagic fevers. I am grateful to him for giving me the opportunity to run the division.

2. Germs as Weapons

1. Jared Diamond, *Guns, Germs, and Steel: The Fates of Human Societies* (New York, W. W. Norton, 1999), 77–78.

2. A. A. Vorobjev et al., "Key Problems of Controlling Especially Dangerous Infections," in *Proceedings of the International Symposium of Severe Infectious Diseases: Epidemiology, Express-Diagnostics and Prevention* (Kirov, Russia: State Scientific Institution, Volgo-Vyatsky Center of Applied Biotechnology, 1997), 71–76.

3. Department of the Army, *U.S. Army Activity in the U.S. Biological Warfare Programs*, vol. 2, *Publication DTIC B193427L* (Washington DC: Department of the Army, 1977).

3. The Six "Chessmen of Doom"

1. In this chapter at the beginning of the section for each "chessman," I list the name of the disease as well as the pathogen that causes the disease. For simplicity, throughout the chapter and elsewhere in the book, I use the name of the disease interchangeably with the pathogen, a common practice in the medical field as well as in lay publications.

2. Zygmunt F. Dembek, Leonard A. Smith, and Janice M. Rusnak, "Botulinum Toxin," in *Textbook of Military Medicine: Medical Aspects of Biological Warfare* (Washington DC: Borden Institute, 2007), 337–53, here 338.

3. Dembek, Smith, and Rusnak, "Botulinum Toxin," 339.

4. World Health Organization Group of Consultants, *Health Aspects of Chemical and Biological Weapons* (Geneva: WHO, 1970).

5. The origins of this nursery rhyme are uncertain. Although it has recently been conjectured to be related to the Black Death, that notion has not been substantiated. David Mikkelson, "Is 'Ring around the Rosie' about the Black Plague?," November 7, 2000, https://www.snopes.com/fact-check/ring-around-rosie/.

6. This affliction is described in various ways after the Philistines moved the ark: "He afflicted the people of the city, both young and old, with an outbreak of tumors." 1 Samuel 5:6 NIV.

7. "Plague—Madagascar," World Health Organization, November 15, 2017, http://www
.who.int/csr/don/15-november-2017-plague-madagascar/en/.

8. Agar, which is derived from seaweed, is a common medium used for growing bacteria. In a process similar to making Jell-O, dried agar is mixed with boiling water and then poured into small glass or plastic petri dishes, where it hardens into a gelatinous substance. Other nutritional or inhibition factors can be mixed in to support or limit the growth of different bacteria or fungi.

4. Hoofbeats

1. USAMRIID commanders were usually colonels, and the commander one level above was a general, who was dual hatted as the Fort Detrick commander and the commanding general of the Medical Research and Materiel Command (MRMC), which had several subordinate laboratories. The commanders had a two- to three-year cycle in charge. During my tenure at USAMRIID, there were five different USAMRIID commanders and four different MRMC commanders, but for the sake of simplicity I have not identified them by name in the narrative.

2. Sadly, John died in December 2015 after a long battle with Parkinson's disease.

3. Rick Weiss and Jo Becker, "Problems in Bioterror Response: First Cases Show Need to Inform Public and Guard against Panic," *Washington Post*, October 14, 2001, A10.

4. Rick Weiss, "Florida Anthrax Case Not a Result of Terrorism, Officials Say," *Washington Post*, October 5, 2001, A15.

5. Streets are named in honor of those victims at Fort Detrick. Another victim who died from Machupo virus infection was also so honored.

5. The Queen Strikes

1. Although I did not provide medical care for O'Connor, I have elected to include only portions from our conversation that were subsequently reported in the media to avoid any potential infringement on O'Connor's medical privacy. The description was derived from the following reports: Michael Powell and Ceci Connolly, "Fourth Case of Anthrax Identified: NBC Employee Tests Positive Weeks after Opening Letter from Fla," *Washington Post*, October 13, 2001, A1; Michael Powell and Justin Blum, "Anthrax Confirmed in 3rd State; Letter from Malaysia Tests Positive in Nev: 2nd NBC Case Possible," *Washington Post*, October 14, 2001, A1.

2. Lawrence K. Altman, "The Doctor's World: When Everything Changed at the C.D.C.," *New York Times*, November 13, 2001, https://www.nytimes.com/2001/11/13/science/the-doctor-s-world-when-everything-changed-at-the-cdc.html.

3. B. Kournikakis et al., *Risk Assessment of Anthrax Threat Letters* Technical Report TR-2001-048 (Suffield AL: Defence Research Establishment Suffield, 2001).

4. Vincent P. Hsu et al., "Opening a Bacillus Anthracis-Containing Envelope, Capitol Hill, Washington DC: The Public Health Response," *Emerging Infectious Diseases* 8, no. 10 (2002): 1039–43.

5. Depending on what someone is working on in the BSL-3 laboratory, and based on a risk assessment, the person may not need to wear additional protective gear if he or she is working in a biological safety cabinet and has been vaccinated against the agent in ques-

tion. Having worked in the Special Pathogens Lab, John no doubt would have been vaccinated against anthrax—numerous times.

6. David Johnston and Alison Mitchell, "A Nation Challenged: The Widening Inquiry; Anthrax Mailed to Senate Is Found to Be Potent Form; Case Tied to Illness at NBC," *New York Times*, October 17, 2001, A00001.

7. Hsu et al., "Opening a Bacillus Anthracis-Containing Envelope."

8. Vahid Majidi, *A Spore on the Grassy Knoll: An Insider's Account of the 2001 Anthrax Mailings* (CreateSpace Independent Publishing Platform, 2013), 39.

6. The Nation's Bio-Emergency Hotline

1. Over this period, which encompasses the U.S. offensive biological weapons program, 439 laboratory infections occurred. The top five included tularemia-153; brucellosis-94; Q fever-55, VEE-43, and anthrax-31.

2. Many engineering features that microbiology labs use today, such as directional airflow, glove boxes, suit labs, and laminar flow hoods, were developed or perfected at Fort Detrick.

3. Autoclaves use a combination of heat, steam, and pressure to sterilize laboratory waste or laboratory and surgical equipment.

7. The Pawn Comes Calling

1. Interview of Condoleezza Rice by George Stephanopoulos, ABC news blog, November 1, 2001, https://www.yahoo.com/news/blogs/abc-blogs/condoleezza-rice-moment -she-thought-president-bush-could-120109212.html.

2. George W. Bush, *Decision Points* (New York: Crown, 2010), 152–53.

3. M. Benjamin, "Biological Alarm in Washington: Did Terrorist Attack Washington with a Deadly Pathogen?," October 18, 2005, http://www.salon.com/2005/10/18/tularemia/.

4. "Tularemia Agent Found in DC Air, but No Cases Seen," CIDRAP News, October 3, 2005, http://www.cidrap.umn.edu/news-perspective/2005/10/tularemia-agent-found -dc-air-no-cases-seen.

8. Bioweapons 101

1. David R. Franz and Nancy K. Jaax, "Ricin Toxin," chap. 32 in *Textbook of Military Medicine: Medical Aspects of Chemical and Biological Warfare* (Washington DC: Borden Institute, 1997), 632–35.

2. Thomas J. Török et al., "A Large Community Outbreak of Salmonellosis Caused by Intentional Contamination of Restaurant Salad Bars," *Journal of the American Medical Association* 278, no. 5 (1997): 389–95.

3. Shellie A. Kolavic et al., "An Outbreak of *Shigella dysenteriae* Type 2 among Laboratory Workers due to Intentional Food Contamination," *Journal of the American Medical Association* 278, no. 5 (1997): 396–98.

4. Mustard agent has an onion, garlic, or mustard odor; lewisite smells like geraniums; and phosgene oxime may smell like newly mown hay.

9. Preparing for Biological Warfare

1. Arthur M. Friedlander et al., "Postexposure Prophylaxis Against Experimental Inhalational Anthrax," *Journal of Infectious Diseases* 167, no. 5 (1993): 1239–42.

2. The request for protocols fell into two tiers, with Tier 1 as first priority:

Diluted (1:5) Smallpox vaccine to prevent smallpox. We had only fifteen million doses for the entire nation of nearly 300 million people, so this would expand the national stockpile.

Vaccinia Immune Globulin, to treat reactions to the smallpox vaccine.

Pentavalent Botulinum toxoid vaccine, to prevent five types of botulism, A through E.

Three types of Botulinum toxin antitoxins, to treat botulism.

Cidofovir—a licensed drug to treat a viral infection, cytomegalovirus, but which would be used to treat smallpox or smallpox vaccine reactions as an IND.

Anthrax vaccine for infants and children

3. Tier 2 included vaccines to prevent the following infections: Q fever, tularemia, VEE, eastern equine encephalitis, western equine encephalitis.

10. Disaster from Within

1. Key physicians at the meeting included Kelly McKee, Phil Pittman, Ellen Boudreau, Patricia Petitt, Scott Stanek, and Mohan Ranadive.

2. Rick Weiss and David Snyder, "2nd Leak of Anthrax Found at Army Lab," *Washington Post,* April 24, 2002, https://www.washingtonpost.com/archive/local/2002/04/24/2nd-leak-of-anthrax-found-at-army-lab/2bb6fd72-b49e-47ab-a4e6-f40ea2e97806/?utm_term=.26e3ce5eb318.

3. To his credit Congressman Bartlett was a longtime champion of the institute and Fort Detrick and was instrumental in arranging a sixtieth anniversary celebration of Fort Detrick's scientific achievements. I had the chance to share the stage with him at another venue as deputy commander several years later honoring the Project White Coat volunteers and have enormous appreciation for his folksy, candid manner.

4. We published a report on these cases in the medical literature; see Janice Rusnak et al., "An Unusual Inhalational Exposure to *Bacillus anthracis* in a Research Laboratory," *Journal of Occupational and Environmental Medicine* 46, no. 4 (2004): 313–14.

5. A CNN report noted, "An employee at the U.S. Army biological lab at Fort Detrick, Maryland, has tested positive for exposure to anthrax, a spokesman said Friday. The employee, who had been previously immunized, is not sick but was put on precautionary antibiotics, base spokesman Chuck Dasey said. Low levels of anthrax spores were found in an administrative room and a service hallway outside a laboratory in one building, Dasey said. Medical assessments of employees were started after a scientist noticed a deposit on a flask in a laboratory where general anthrax research is conducted, he said." Kevin Bohn, "Fort Detrick Worker Exposed to Anthrax," April 19, 2002, http://www.cnn.com/2002/US/04/19/fort.detrick.anthrax/index.html.

Another report from the University of Minnesota's CIDRAP stated: "The sampling and testing were triggered when a scientist noticed a deposit on a flask in the lab on Apr 8, according to the Army." Robert Roos, "Anthrax Escapes Lab Room at USAMRIID; One Worker Exposed," CIDRAP News, April 23, 2002, www.cidrap.umn.edu/news-perspective/2002/04/anthrax-escapes-lab-room-usamriid-one-worker-exposed.

6. A redacted report of the 15–6 investigation, titled "AR 15–6 Investigation into Anthrax Contamination at USAMRIID," May 16, 2001, is available at https://www.documentcloud.org/documents/89814-h4-usamriid-ba-contamination-ar-15-6.

11. Bow to King Smallpox

1. Edward Jenner, "The Origin of the Vaccine Inoculation" (London: D. N. Shury, 1801), cited by Andreas Aly and Sophia Aly, Letter, *New England Journal of Medicine* 335, no. 12 (1996): 900–902.

2. USAMRIID investigators led much of the new research on smallpox countermeasures, but they could not work on the virus at USAMRIID due to international treaty restrictions. The CDC was the only place in the United States allowed to possess the virus; therefore our investigators had to conduct their work there.

3. Every organization in the military has a "chain of command." USAMRIID fell under a large command, the MRMC. USAMRIID was just one of several research institutes that fell under the MRMC. The MRMC's headquarters was within a couple of blocks of USAMRIID, on Fort Detrick.

12. On the Front Lines

1. As of 2016 178 nations had signed the convention. Six more have signed it but have not yet ratified the treaty.

2. We call this "SLUDGE:" salivation, lacrimation, urination, diaphoresis (sweating), gastrointestinal upset (including diarrhea), emesis (vomiting).

3. Department of Defense Directive 3216.2 (March 25, 2002) describes the protection of human subjects and adherence to ethical standards in DoD-supported research. Paragraph 2.3 of this directive notes that the directive "does not apply to the use of investigational new drugs, biological products, or devices for purposes of Force Health Protection. Such use is not research and is governed by DoD Directive 6200.2." The difficulty in knowing what standard to reference is that products used for treatment, such as botulinum antitoxin or vaccinia immune globulin, *are* the standard of care and at the time had to be given under a research protocol specifically for force health protection and treatment.

Meeting all the requirements of the FDA in a war environment is an extremely high bar. The BIG (human) product, originally intended as an intravenous treatment protocol, had to be changed to an intramuscular prevention protocol due to the FDA's concerns about increased protein aggregates that had developed in the product over time.

4. SMART-IND members (members deploying with me italicized):

> Doctors: Edwin Anderson, Phil Coyne, Timothy Endy, *Donald Gray Heppner*, Niranjan Kanesa-thasan, Kent Kester, *Mark Kortepeter, Robert Kuschner, Alan Magill, Christian Ockenhouse*, Bret Purcell
>
> Nurses: *Jackie Carlin*, Mishelle Morris-Magee
>
> Noncommissioned Officers: SFC *Marc Schenker*, SGT *Henderson*, SGT *Hall*
>
> Medical Service Corps Officers: *Colleen Martinez*, Isaiah (Ike) Harper, Jeffrey Gere

Other staff providing support to the SMART-IND team effort included Arthur Anderson, Ellen Boudreau, John Huggins, Laura Brosch, MG (RET) Lester Martinez-Lopez, Judy Pace, Patricia Petitt, Jerry Pierson, Philip Pittman, and Manmohan Ranadive.

I am particularly grateful to my deploying team members Alan Magill, Gray Heppner, and Chris Ockenhouse, as well as others on the team who didn't deploy (Bret Purcell, Kent Kester, Tim Endy), and Jim Cummings for encouraging me to apply for an infectious disease fellowship after the deployment and to join the infectious disease community.

5. "Bill" is a pseudonym for a colleague from the intelligence community.

13. Desert Pneumonia

1. Janice did a phone interview with *Washington Post* writer Dr. David Brown about this outbreak. I was supposed to join in the call but was pulled away for other meetings, so Janice did it alone. Although I have my own memory of the events and my later discussions with Janice, this article also helped tease my memory.

I am noted anonymously in the article in two places (italicized here): "First, he [Dr. Bruno Petruccelli] received a copy of several e-mails Rusnak had sent from Germany to *colleagues* at the Army's infectious disease research center at Fort Detrick in Frederick," and "Shortly after he had read both messages, Petruccelli got a call from *the doctor* at Fort Detrick who had forwarded Rusnak's emails. *He* wanted to talk about them." As Dr. Petruccelli is quoted in the article: "You couldn't have done it better in Hollywood. It all kind of blows in one day." David Brown, "Troops' Pneumonia Outbreak Spurs Medical Hunt," *Washington Post*, September 12, 2003, A1.

2. A. L. Korenyi-Both, A. C. Molnár, and R. Fidelus-Gort, "Al Eskan Disease: Desert Storm Pneumonitis," *Military Medicine* 157, no. 9 (1992): 452–62.

3. Andrew F. Shorr et al., "Acute Eosinophilic Pneumonia among U.S. Military Personnel Deployed in or near Iraq," *Journal of the American Medical Association* 293, no. 24 (2004): 2997–3005.

14. The 4M Disaster

1. Brian Susi et al., "Rapid Diagnostic Test for *Plasmodium falciparum* in 32 Marines Medically Evacuated from Liberia with a Febrile Illness," *Annals of Internal Medicine*, 142, no. 6, (2005): 476–77.

2. A Medical Board is a formal summary describing a military person's illness and medical course, similar to a hospital discharge note. In the past, if a soldier died while on active duty, his or her family's benefits would be limited, but if the soldier were "medically retired" with a fully dictated medical board before he or she died, the family received more military benefits after the death. Hence, when someone was dying, dictating the board before death was an urgent matter. The rules have changed, so this is no longer required.

3. Communication between military infectious disease officers across the world was facilitated for years by an annual meeting of the Armed Forces Infectious Disease Society, a subgroup under the Infectious Disease Society of America. Unfortunately, the funds to continue this valuable professional interface are now limited, and new military rules have

curtailed interactions with civilian counterparts, which means a huge loss of this collaboration venue.

4. Timothy J. Whitman et al., "An Outbreak of *Plasmodium falciparum* Malaria in U.S. Marines Deployed to Liberia," *American Journal of Tropical Medicine and Hygiene* 83, no. 2 (2010): 258–65.

15. Countermeasures

1. The biodefense program has developed numerous vaccines and vaccine candidates against tularemia, Q fever, Rift Valley fever virus, Junin virus, 3 equine encephalitis viruses, Staphylococcal enterotoxin B, chikungunya, plague, smallpox, Ebola, hantaviruses, ricin, botulism, and others.

16. The Slammer

1. Meeting participants included Larry Lepler (ICU doctor from Walter Reed who led the critical care team), Jim Martin (infectious disease doctor who served as the patient's primary physician), Mark Kortepeter (preventive medicine doctor and Medicine Division chief), Scott Stanek (chief of the Operational Medicine Division who "owned" the Slammer facility), Bret Purcell (infectious disease doctor and bacteriology researcher), Ed Anderson (pediatric infectious disease doctor and assistant chief of Medicine Division), Ellen Boudreau (chief of the Special Immunizations Program in the clinic and first physician to see the patient after the exposure), Ben Woods (pediatric infectious disease doctor in Operational Medicine Division), Tony Littrell (preventive medicine doctor in Operational Medicine Division), Matt Hepburn (infectious disease doctor in Medical Division), Alan Schmaljohn (virologist), C. J. Peters (physician/scientist from University of Texas, Galveston), Peter Jahrling (USAMRIID senior scientist), Karl Johnson (physician/tropical virologist), Pierre Rollin (physician/epidemiologist at the CDC), Heinz Feldmann (physician/scientist at Health Canada's containment lab), Art Anderson (physician/pathologist/ethicist at USAMRIID), Eric Henchal (scientist and USAMRIID commander), Sandra Flynn (Operational Medicine Division secretary), Tom Geisbert (USAMRIID virologist), and Sina Bavari (USAMRIID scientist).

2. Sina later became USAMRIID's senior scientist.

3. When scientists grow viruses in cell culture, they can estimate virus concentrations by observing abnormalities in a monolayer of the cells called "plaques." A single "plaque forming unit" is considered evidence of growth of the virus in the cell culture. Dianne is implying that even a single virus particle of Ebola could be enough to kill.

4. Phil W. Smith et al., "Designing a Biocontainment Unit to Care for Patients with Serious Communicable Diseases: A Consensus Statement," *Biosecurity and Bioterrorism* 24, no. 4 (2006): 351–65.

5. Mark G. Kortepeter et al., "Managing Potential Laboratory Exposure to Ebola Virus by Using a Patient Biocontainment Care Unit," *Emerging Infectious Diseases* 14, no. 6 (2008): 881–87.

17. On the Hot Side

1. I picked up an unfinished study that my colleagues Rob Rivard and James Lawler had begun. Like any research study, completing it requires a team of individuals. I was grate-

ful for the assistance of my lab colleagues Anna Honko, Gene Olinger, Joshua Johnson, Keith Esham, and Lisa Hensley. Rob, James, Bret Purcell, and Matt Hepburn also assisted with monitoring the animals during the disease course. Mike Bray provided much assistance in writing the article.

2. Despite its popularity with the public, we don't typically use the term *hot zone* to describe the containment laboratory environment. Using *sides* instead has much more practical meaning: we can immediately pinpoint where someone is working and his or her potential risks if exposure occurs. The "hot" side refers to the section of the lab where we work directly with disease agents or infected animals, and the "cold" side is free from such risks. The "warm" side is an area between the two. At USAMRIID the "hot" labs are configured as a series of smaller laboratories or animal rooms, with their own doors, on both sides of a central corridor. This group of labs, collectively, make up a "hot suite," with a single entrance and exit.

The process for getting authorized to enter a containment lab is long and involved— with vetting by security staff, safety training, training in biological surety, regulations, working with animals, and so on. The whole process can take up to a year.

Generally, we prefer to have people work in the BSL-2 or BSL-3 laboratories before working in BSL-4. This provides time for observing someone's safety practices where there is lower risk before moving to the next level. The last thing we want is an employee getting an extended "vacation" in the Slammer.

3. Autoclave tape is very similar to masking tape and is used in an operating room to tape down cloth holding surgical instruments. It has stripes on it that change color, indicating whether the material is pre- or post-autoclave.

4. There are several reasons for requiring this final barrier to the hot side. First, if an unauthorized person manages to access this far into the lab, it provides a final security barrier. Second, it provides an electronic time stamp of who entered and exited (and when). Third, if someone is working alone on the hot side, security personnel can pull up the entry log and see who remains in containment.

5. Mark G. Kortepeter et al., "Real-Time Monitoring of Cardiovascular Function in Rhesus Macaques Infected with *Zaire ebolavirus,*" *Journal of Infectious Diseases* 204, no. S3 (2011): S1000–1010.

19. Suspicion

1. K. Heerbrandt, "A Shocking Mockery," *Frederick News Post*, August 12, 2009.

20. The Aftermath

1. Pat Worsham's eulogy follows:

When I came to USAMRIID as a new PI, I was welcomed into the division by Bruce with great enthusiasm. We shared an office, along with our technicians Michelle Sowers and Pat Fellows. Bruce made a point of acquainting me in great detail with Frederick and USAMRIID. He was the one who made me feel at home. In these early years, we shared in that office and in our labs many hours of scientific discussions, political debate, and gossip. Bruce had a vibrant, active mind. He was never boring. Over the years Bacteriology developed a well-deserved reputation for cohesiveness, exuberance, and team spirit. We truly enjoy one another's company. Bruce was a big part of that.

Bruce was always the first to express condolences, the first to offer a hug when there was a sad event in someone's life. If I were frazzled and rushing about with no time to talk to him I would come back to find a pack (or two) of peanut M and Ms on my desk. He knew my weakness. I wish I could share with you all of the poems and songs he wrote over the years for various occasions. He was incredibly clever, articulate, and sensitive. He had a beautiful voice.

The thing we learned to avoid were the pun-fests between Bruce and John Ezzell.

I recently found out that Monica O'Guinn and I had a common and somewhat embarrassing secret: we both watched *Survivor*, and we really looked forward to discussing the episodes in detail with Bruce on Fridays.

Beyond his science that Bret and Art described, the great and lasting contribution of Bruce's is his mentorship of the next generation of scientists. Young people from his lab moved on, with his nurturing and encouragement, to graduate school, medical school, and positions of greater professional responsibility. He purposefully yielded the limelight so that they could have the opportunity to discuss and present their work as primary authors. He was always generous and selfless with his time and his knowledge.

One of his enduring gifts sits in the audience today: Anthony Bassett was a soldier in Veterinary Medicine here at USAMRIID and found himself at a crossroads. If he left the army, USAMRIID had a number of PIs interested in hiring him. If he stayed in service, he would be moving on to new and exciting frontiers. Bruce recognized Anthony's potential and convinced him to come to Bacteriology. For Anthony this was a major turning point in his life. As a result Anthony met his wife, Jennifer, and they started their home and lives together. And from a selfish point of view, he became an invaluable institute resource. This is part of Bruce's legacy sitting right here with us.

We all want to thank Bruce for his scientific contributions, his enthusiasm, and his friendship.

2. William J. Broad and Scott Shane, "Scientists' Analysis Disputes FBI Closing of Anthrax Case," *New York Times*, October 9, 2001, A1.

3. Dugway Proving Ground is a military research and testing facility in Utah where some outdoor bioweapons testing in the army's offensive bioweapons program was conducted.

4. Carrie Johnson, Del Quentin Wilber, and Dan Eggen, "Government Asserts Ivins Acted Alone," *Washington Post*, August 7, 2008, A1.

5. Susan Welkos et al., "Bruce Edwards Ivins," *Microbe* 3, no. 11 (2008): 542.

6. Jerry Markon, "Case Turns the Justice Department on Itself," *Washington Post*, January 29, 2012, A3.

7. Scott Shane, "Former FBI Agent Sues, Claiming Retaliation over Misgivings in Anthrax Case," *New York Times*, April 9, 2015, A21.

21. Down for the Count

1. Associated Press, "Iraq Got Seeds for Bioweapons from U.S.," *Baltimore Sun*, October 1, 2002. https://www.baltimoresun.com/news/nation-world/bal-te.bioweapons01oct01-story.html.

2. Federal Select Agent Program, "Select Agents and Toxins List," accessed August 11, 2018, https://www.selectagents.gov/selectagentsandtoxinslist.html.

3. Nuclear "surety" programs have been in place for decades to ensure the safety and security of nuclear devices and workers involved with them. Similar programs had also been adopted for chemical warfare agents (nerve agents, blister agents, etc.). The programs for biological agents were not as well formed until recently, although various infractions over time led to increasing restrictions and policies, primarily on transfer of agents from one location to another. Much of what governed use of the agents had already been in place through CDC and NIH guidance on laboratory safety by categorizing agents into specific biological safety levels, BSL-1 through BSL-4. The guidance on use and transfer of agents of concern for bioterrorism and major public health disasters falls under what is called the "Select Agent" program run by the CDC.

The DoD made significant changes after 2001 in an analogous program called "biosurety." This included a combination of maintaining security of the organisms themselves (the agents), and safety of the workforce. There are four basic pillars: enhancing safety, security measures, personnel reliability, and agent accountability. The institute always had a very robust safety program, as evidenced by an admirable track record of worker safety over decades, which hasn't changed even since 2001, in addition to excellent containment of agents in the laboratories. Procedures have evolved significantly since 2001, mostly in the latter three pillars.

After the FBI's accusations about Bruce Ivins, the army responded with its own set of new guidelines (although some might call them punishments). In 2001, when the army mandated several changes in the other three pillars, they seemed stringent at the time. In retrospect many of the measures were reasonable and ahead of their time.

As far as personnel reliability, the army sought to institute a program that mirrored what had already been in place for years in the nuclear and chemical arenas. This was a major undertaking for USAMRIID, as there were over 250 people in the institute who had to be inducted into the program. Prior to 9/11 USAMRIID's Special Immunization Program (SIP) had its own way of weeding out individuals who wouldn't fare well in the containment laboratories based on medical problems or health requirements for vaccination with investigational vaccines. Individuals also underwent national agency law-enforcement checks.

With the addition of the Personnel Reliability Program (PRP), individuals now had to undergo local and national agency checks, had to submit to random drug testing, and be "read into" the program. Once they are in the program, if they see a doctor, get a new prescription, go bankrupt, or have a run-in with the law, they must bring this to the attention of their certifying official (CO). If they don't report the items mentioned above in their initial interview or along the way, they can be deemed "unreliable" and removed from the program. Despite initial misgivings, the workforce generally adapted to the program without too much difficulty. We did finally get everyone enrolled, but the requirement continues to be a significant burden. Also the PRP adds a barrier to collaboration because it is stricter than comparable measures at other research organizations and imposes restrictions on working with those that do not have a similar program.

4. William B Genougreh III, "Update on Dr. Thomas Butler," *Clinical Infectious Diseases* 43, no. 2 (2006): 259–60. The case of Thomas Butler provides a cautionary note regarding the risk of working with select agents for anyone in the scientific field, especially in the highly charged post-9/11 era.

5. In February 2009 the army sent out a formal message called an ALARACT in military-speak—meaning "all army activities" should take notice.

6. The need to create this database came from a new code of federal regulations requirement. The institute inventoried its agent database regularly and was subject to regular inspections by the Department of the Army Inspector General (DAIG), in addition to the CDC and other authorities.

7. The extra four vials of VEE were probably original isolates used to make more vials of organisms for experiments but were never entered into the database.

8. Yudhijit Bhattacharjee, "Army Halts Work at Lab after Finding Untracked Material," *Science* 323, no. 5916 (2009): 861.

9. This comment is a more succinct version of a remark by German military strategist Helmut von Moltke that has previously been attributed to Eisenhower. Moltke's original observation in the mid-nineteenth century was "No operation extends with any certainty beyond the first encounter with the main body of the enemy." Ralph Keyes, "The Quote Verifier: Who Said What, Where, and When," accessed October 12, 2018, https://ralphkeyes.com/book/quote-verifier/.

10. Bhattacharjee, "Army Halts Work."

11. Ironically, Sam is now the CDC's head for select agent accountability, making him now the enforcer of the rules he had to follow.

12. The big mistake I made was accepting a follow-up interview with the same *Science* reporter who had done the original report. I felt like he was gunning for us, repeatedly asking me whether we were in violation with the Code of Federal Regulations. See Yudhijit Bhattacharjee, "Discovery of Untracked Pathogen Vials at Army Lab Sparks Concerns," *Science* 324, no. 5935 (2009): 1626.

13. Over time the institute had been moved from a government funding model, where it had a set amount of funds channeled to the Institute annually, to an academic model, based on proposals submitted by investigators. The Defense Threat Reduction Agency (DTRA) was the primary funder but would no longer guarantee USAMRIID its usual funding at a time when numerous other containment labs were being built across the country and universities also began competing for funds. This unnecessarily pitted scientists against one another in the proposal process and also led to some scientific departments reaping huge benefits while others were left to pick up residual crumbs.

14. Bhattacharjee, "Discovery of Untracked Pathogen Vials."

15. Brady Dennis and Lena H. Sun, "FDA Found More Than Smallpox Vials in Storage Room," *Washington Post*, July 16, 2014, https://www.washingtonpost.com/national/health-science/fda-found-more-than-smallpox-vials-in-storage-room/2014/07/16/850d4b12-0d22-11e4-8341-b8072b1e7348_story.html?utm_term=.5cb3c54de4a4.

22. Behind the Scenes of Pandemic Response

1. Colonel James Cummings, R&D consultant to the army surgeon general; Colonel Stephen Thomas, ID consultant to the army surgeon general, and I, as consultant to the army surgeon general for biodefense, sent these summaries up the chain of command weekly.

2. I signed the memo, dated August 27, 2014, to the Pentagon under the subject line: "Deployable DoD Clinical Care Packages: Response to the W. Africa Ebola Outbreak."

The consensus team included a who's who of senior military infectious disease leaders at the time: Colonel James Cummings, R&D consultant to the army surgeon general; Colonel Stephen Thomas, ID consultant to the army surgeon general; Colonel Mark Kortepeter, biodefense consultant to the army surgeon general; Captain David Blazes, navy specialty leader for ID; Lieutenant Colonel Nick Conger, ID consultant to the air force surgeon general; Commander James Lawler, Naval Medical Research Center; and Commander David Brett-Major, seconded to WHO.

3. Lena H. Sun, "Official: U.S. Military's Response to Ebola Hampered by Lack of Expertise with Virus," *Washington Post*, September 9, 2014, italics added, https://www .washingtonpost.com/national/health-science/official-us-response-to-ebola-hampered-by -lack-of-expertise-with-deadly-virus/2014/09/09/343e5cd8-385d-11e4-9c9f-ebb47272e40e _story.html?utm_term=.bd7b7c1c443e.

4. Commander David Brett-Major had been working at the WHO headquarters in Geneva as a military liaison before the outbreak began. Consequently, as a "seconded" asset, he was sent to West Africa and cared for numerous patients in Sierra Leone and Nigeria. He wrote a book describing his experience: David M. Brett-Major, *A Year of Ebola: A Personal Tale of the Weirdness Wrought by the World's Largest Ebola Virus Disease Epidemic* (Bethesda MD: Navigating Health Risks, 2016). Commander James Lawler was able to get to Guinea for a short stint before the DoD closed the door.

5. Randall J. Schoepp et al., "Undiagnosed Acute Viral Febrile Illnesses, Sierra Leone," *Emerging Infectious Diseases* 20, no. 7 (2014): 1176–82.

6. Dr. Brantley was the first Ebola victim from the large 2014–16 outbreak in West Africa who was brought to the United States for care.

7. ZMapp is a cocktail of three monoclonal antibodies developed from early research efforts at USAMRIID and the Canadian biodefense lab. Xiangguo Qiu et al., "Reversion of Advanced Ebola Virus Disease in Nonhuman Primates with ZMapp," *Nature* 514, no. 2 (October 2014): 47–53.

8. Mark G. Kortepeter, et al., "Containment Care Units for Managing Patients with Highly Hazardous Infectious Diseases: A Concept Whose Time Has Come," *Journal of Infectious Diseases* 214, no. S3 (2016): S137–41.

9. Mark G. Kortepeter et al., "Caring for Ebola Patients: A Challenge in Any Care Facility, *Annals of Internal Medicine* 162, no. 1 (2015): 68–69.

10. Amy B. Adler et al., "Quarantine and the U.S. Military Response to the Ebola Crisis: Soldier Health and Attitudes," *Public Health* 155 (2018): 95–98.

11. PREVAIL II Writing Group, "A Randomized, Controlled Trial of ZMapp for Ebola Virus Infection," *New England Journal of Medicine* 375, no. 15 (2016): 1448–56.

12. J. R. Spengler et al., "Management of a Pet Dog after Exposure to a Human Patient with Ebola Virus Disease," *Journal of the American Veterinary Association* 247, no. 5 (2015): 531–38.

13. The agencies include individual country ministries of health, WHO, the CDC, MSF, NIAID, the DoD, the State Department, and others.

23. Looking Forward—the Challenges Continue

1. Elizabeth Philipp, Hyun-Kyung Kim, and Hattie Chung, "North Korea's Biological Weapons Program: The Known and Unknown," Belfer Center for Science and Inter-

national Affairs, Harvard Kennedy School, October 2017, https://www.belfercenter.org/publication/north-koreas-biological-weapons-program-known-and-unknown.

2. Ken Alibek, *Biohazard: The Chilling True Story of the Largest Covert Biological Weapons Program in the World—Told from Inside by the Man Who Ran It* (New York: Dell, 1999).

3. R. Grunow and E.-J. Finke, "A Procedure for Differentiating between the Intentional Release of Biological Warfare Agents and Natural Outbreaks of Disease: Its Use in Analyzing the Tularemia Outbreak in Kosovo in 1999 and 2000," *Clinical Microbiology and Infection* 8, no. 8 (2002): 510–21.

4. Zygmunt F. Dembek, Mark G. Kortepeter, and Julie A. Pavlin, "Discernment between Deliberate and Natural Infectious Disease Outbreaks," *Epidemiology and Infection* 135, no. 3 (2007): 353–71.

5. I met Dr. Folk and learned about his experience when he gave a lecture to the NATO Biomedical Advisory Panel at one of our meetings.

6. Larry M. Bush and Maria T. Perez, "The Anthrax Attacks 10 Years Later," *Annals of Internal Medicine* 156, no. 1 (2012): 41–44.

Carlin, Jackie, 114, 258n4

Casals, Jordi, 135–36

category A threat agents: 14–15, 234. *See also* anthrax; botulinum toxin; Ebola virus; Lassa fever virus; Marburg virus; plague; smallpox; tularemia; viral hemorrhagic fevers

CCHF. *See* Crimean Congo hemorrhagic fever

CDC. *See* Centers for Disease Control and Prevention

Centers for Disease Control and Prevention (CDC): botulinum antitoxins available at, 56, 62; category A threat list, 15; and discovery of Heartland virus, 240–41; and discovery of Lassa virus, 130, 136; Ebola discovery and, 19–20; and Ebola-infected dogs, 230–32; Erin O'Conner skin biopsy, 37; response to anthrax attacks, 31, 33, 73–74, 88; response to Ebola exposure, 151, 154, 160; response to positive air samplers, 63; select agents and, 203–5, 214, 218–19; September 11, 2001, and, 29; smallpox repository at, 71, 92; and smallpox vaccination, 93, 96; and West Africa Ebola outbreak response, 221, 223, 225–27

chain of command, USAMRIID, 258n3

chemical weapons: 12–13, 17, 70, 100–102, 119; Aum Shinrikyo use of, 65–66; and B'nai B'rith hoax, 68, properties of, 70–72, 256n4; "SLUDGE" nerve agent effects of, 258n2. *See also* mustard blister agent; sarin nerve agent; Soman nerve agent; Tabun nerve agent; VX nerve agent

Cheney, Richard "Dick": and botulinum exposures, 62; and smallpox preparedness, 93, 95, 98; and SMART-IND team, 105

Chessmen, 14–27. *See also* anthrax; botulism; Ebola virus; Lassa fever virus; Marburg virus; plague; smallpox; tularemia; viral hemorrhagic fevers

chikungunya, 143, 260n1

Christie, Chris, 228

CID. *See* criminal investigation division

Cieslak, Ted, 10, 27

Clizbe, Denise, xxiii, 39–40, 162–63

Clostridium botulinum. See botulinum toxin

"cold" side, xvii, 80, 167, 198, 210

combat support hospital (CSH): Eighty-Sixth CSH, 111–14; Twenty-Eighth CSH, 123–24

Comfort hospital ship, 117–19

Conger, Nick, 264–65n2

Cook, Robin, 34

Coyne, Phil, 258n4

Crichton, Michael: *The Andromeda Strain* (book), xxi, 253n1

Crimean Congo hemorrhagic fever (CCHF) virus, 216–17

criminal investigation division (CID), 206–7

CSH. *See* combat support hospital

Cummings, James "Jim," 258–59n4, 264–65nn1–2

Dallas Presbyterian Hospital, 227, 231

Daschle, Tom, 39–43, 45, 51, 88, 177

Dasey, Chuck, 160, 257n5

Defense Threat Reduction Agency (DTRA), 264n3

Defraites, Bob, 125–26, 138

Demmin, Gretchen, 176–77

Department of Defense Ebola working group, 221–23

desert pneumonia, 122–28

Deye, Greg, 134–35, 137

Doctors Without Borders. *See* Médecins Sans Frontières (MSF)

DTRA. *See* Defense Threat Reduction Agency

Dugway Proving Ground, 199, 262n3

Duncan, Thomas, 227, 231

dunk tank, 81

eastern equine encephalitis virus, 75, 257n3

Eastwood, Clint, 80

Ebola virus: biocontainment care for, 226–27; as a biological weapon, 15, 19–21, 69–70; as a BSL-4 pathogen, 49; clinical features of, xix, xxiv, 19, 69, 130, 148–49, 158–59; dog infection with, 229–32; false alarm, 28; fear of infection from, 21, 68; future research on, 172, 236, 308; history of discovery, 19–20, 154; in *The Hot Zone* book, xiii, 154, 253n3; Kelly Warfield work on, xvii–xix; mouse adapted, 264n6; outbreak preparation, 235; pathophysiology studies on, 165–72; Slammer aftermath from, 164; soldier quarantine for, 228–29; USAMRIID response to lab exposure from, xx–xxvi, 146–64; West Africa outbreak of, 12, 129, 142, 145, 220–29

Staphylococcal enterotoxin B (SEB), 143,
  260n1
Starbucks, 115, 149, 151–52, 157
Stephanopoulos, George, 62
Stevens, Robert, 30–33, 38, 201
Streptococcus pneumoniae, 4–5
Sudan, 19–20
Sverdlovsk, Soviet Union, 74
Swearengen, Jim, 254n5

Tabun nerve agent, 71
Tasker, Sybil, 134, 136, 140
task force (Pentagon), 196–97, 208
Thomas, Stephen, 228–29, 264–65nn1–2
Thompson, Dianne, 67–68, 240
Thompson, Tommy, 18, 30
Tripler Army Medical Center (Hawaii), 7–9
Trump administration, 234
tuberculosis, 20, 35, 49
tularemia: airborne alert, 63; as a bioweapon
  agent, 13, 15, 18–19, 70, 240, 243; clinical features of, 18, 35; lab-acquired infection from, 47, 237–39, 256n1; and marine
  fever outbreak, 125; source in nature, 70;
  USAMRIID research on, xx, 143–44, 243;
  war preparation for, 75
typhoid, 20, 25, 66
typhus, 35, 126

Uniformed Services University (USU), 141,
  219, 221, 246
Unit 731, 23
United States Army Medical Unit (USAMU),
  47, 143
University of Nebraska Medical Center and
  College of Public Health, 163–64, 226–
  27, 246
University of Texas, 244, 260
USS *Iwo Jima* Amphibious Ready Group, 129–
  31, 133–34

Vander Linden, Caree, 150, 160, 191, 193, 212–13
variolation, 24, 91–92
variola virus. *See* smallpox
Vaxicools, 108, 109, 112
Venezuelan equine encephalitis (VEE), 206–8,
  256n1, 264n7
vice president. *See* Cheney, Richard
Vicker's unit, 225

violin, 2, 106, 174
viral hemorrhagic fevers, 15, 19–21, 68, 225.
  See also Ebola virus; hantavirus pulmonary syndrome; Junin virus; Lassa fever
  virus; Machupo virus; Marburg; Rift Valley fever virus
Von Moltke, Helmut, 264n9
VX nerve agent, 17, 71, 102, 234

Walter Reed Army Institute of Research
  (WRAIR), 9, 86, 97
Walter Reed Army Medical Center, 118, 124,
  156–57, 165, 226
Warfield, Kelly: Ebola exposure, xvii–xviii,
  xix–xx, xxii–xxiv, 145; Slammer admission
  decision, xxiv–xxvi; Slammer quarantine,
  146–64, 254n7
"warm" side, xvii, xx, 167
western equine encephalitis virus, 75, 257n3
West Nile virus, 50, 217
wheat stem rust, 14
White Coat Program, 143, 144, 257n3
White House: anthrax attack and, 88; bio-
  defense needs, 50, 237; botulinum toxin
  attack and, 51–63; Iraq war and, 75, 93, 98
WHO. *See* World Health Organization
Willman, David, 192
Wine, Laura, 130
Winkenwerder, William, 74, 76–78, 105–6
Wise, Robert: *The Andromeda Strain* (movie),
  49, 225
Wolcott, Mark, 231–32
Woods, Ben, 260n1
World Health Organization (WHO), 25, 92, 221
World Trade Center, 29, 33
Worsham, Pat: aftermath of Ivins death, 192,
  194, 202; anthrax spore characterization
  and, 42, 198–99; FBI investigation and,
  178–81, 185, 187–88; and Ivins arrest, 176–
  77; Ivins eulogy by, 261–62n1
Wyeth Pharmaceuticals, 94, 98, 103

Yale University, 130, 135–36
Yersinia pestis. See plague

Zaire, xxiv, 19–21, 154, 254n6
Zika virus, 12, 145, 235
ZMapp, 224, 229, 265n7